DIVING INJURIES

Research Findings and Recommendations for Reducing Catastrophic Injuries

M. Alexander Gabrielsen, Ph.D.
James McElhaney, Ph.D.
Ron O'Brien, Ph.D.

CRC Press
Boca Raton   London   New York   Washington, D.C.

Cover photograph: Diver interacting with the upslope of a pool's bottom as indicated by the dotted line at a depth of four feet. The photograph was taken at Nova Southeastern University's Dive/Slide Research Pool in Ft. Lauderdale, Florida.

Library of Congress Cataloging-in-Publication Data

Gabrielsen, M. Alexander.
    Diving injuries : research findings and recommendations for reducing catastrophic injuries / M. Alexander Gabrielsen, James McElhaney, Ron O'Brien.
        p. cm.
    Includes bibliographical references and index.
    ISBN 0-8493-2370-3 (alk. paper)
        1. Diving accidents. 2. Swimming pools—Accidents. 3. Swimming pools—Safety measures I. McElhaney, James. II. O'Brien, Ronald F. III. Title.

    RC1220.D5 G33 2000
    617.1′027—dc21   00-03970

Preface

Diving, without question, is the most exciting and challenging activity associated with water; yet diving produces more quadriplegics than all other sports combined. Today there are an estimated 19,000 people sitting in wheelchairs as a result of breaking their necks when diving. I have spent the last 30 years studying the diving injury problem in the United States. This book contains the most comprehensive study of data related to diving injuries. It reports on 440 cases that occurred in swimming pools and 161 that occurred in water areas located in the natural environment.

The primary purpose of this book is to provide the public; governmental agencies; and those who design, plan, engineer, manufacture, sell, construct, regulate, own, and operate swimming pools and swimming beaches with essential information that I believe can enable them to perform their duties and functions with greater understanding and knowledge of the problem of safety as it relates to diving. It is further hoped that the publication will serve as a challenge to the thousands of swimming and diving instructors, teachers, and coaches to place greater emphasis on safety in their instructional programs. Everyone associated with aquatics, including owners of home pools, needs to reflect on the data contained in this book and the recommendations set forth by the authors.

Readers must not interpret the conclusions and recommendations in any way as an indictment of diving or swimming pools. Competitive divers sustain very few injuries. To date, there is no record of any competitive diver receiving a neck fracture by striking the bottom of a pool that met the specifications promulgated by the various ruling bodies governing competitive diving. As the data in this book reveal, the recreational diver is at greatest risk.

Swimming pools represent one of the greatest boons to family living and recreation. They are the safest place to swim but, in the opinion of the authors, they can be made safer and can be operated in a manner that would significantly reduce the number of diving injuries and drownings that occur each year in pools. Chapter 9 addresses injuries that occurred in bodies of water found in the natural environment, such as lakes, rivers, ponds, streams, quarries, and oceans.

The data presented are undeniable. On the other hand, the conclusions and recommendations are the opinions of the authors based on the data recorded in this book, their many years of teaching swimming and diving, and the years of research that they have conducted relative to diving injuries. There will be some who may disagree with our recommendations, particularly our decision not to entirely exclude diving into the shallow portion of pools as outlined in Chapter 15, "The Dilemma".

We sense very keenly the need to continue research in the area. Many critical questions remain unanswered—questions that have direct consequences for a theoretical system that permits scientifically accurate comparison of prediction with experience. Today, enough is now known; and the place, person, and injury frequency are so predictable that action toward accident prevention must begin at once.

M. Alexander Gabrielsen, Ph.D.
Fort Lauderdale, Florida

Authors

M. Alexander Gabrielsen, Ph.D. is Professor Emeritus of New York University (NYU) where he served from 1946 to 1970. While at NYU, he developed and headed the professional curriculum in the field of recreation and camping. He has authored and co-authored 15 books and many professional articles on sports and recreation facilities. Dr. Gabrielsen, serving in the Navy during World War II and the Korean and Vietnam Wars, was promoted to Captain in 1960. He has been a consultant to foreign countries, colleges, universities, cities, and schools in the United States on the planning of swimming pools.

Dr. Gabrielsen was affiliated with Nova University (now Nova Southeastern) from 1972 until 1985 as Special Assistant to the President. It was at that time that he created the Nova Dive/Slide Research Center. Dr. Gabrielsen has conducted research on all forms of diving and sliding (springboard/jumpboard dives from starting blocks and from pool decks). He conducted studies for the Consumer Product Safety Commission (CPSC) on water slides and diving boards, and collected data on diving accidents occurring in swimming pools.

Dr. Gabrielsen was a competitive swimmer and diver in high school and college. He coached high school and college students, Boys' Club members, and four girls who broke 34 national and 7 world records. In his lifetime he has taught thousands of youngsters and adults to swim and dive.

James H. McElhaney, Ph.D. is the Hudson Distinguished Professor of Biomechanics in the Departments of Biomedical Engineering and Orthopaedic Surgery, Duke University. He is former chairman of the Department of Biomechanical Engineering (1983 to 1995). He is a fellow of the Institute for Engineering in Medicine and Biology and the American Society of Mechanical Engineers. He is the author of over 170 papers on injury biomechanics and three books including the *Handbook of Human Tolerance*. He has received the John Paul Stapp Award five times for the best biomechanics paper at the annual Stapp Car Crash Conference. Prior to his appointment at Duke University, he was the head of the Biomechanics Department at the Highway Safety Research Institute of the University of Michigan. His primary research interest is the biomechanical aspects of head and neck injury. He received his Ph.D. from West Virginia University.

Ron O'Brien, Ph.D. has been involved in aquatics for over 50 years as an athlete, teacher, and coach. He received his Ph.D. from The Ohio State University. Dr. O'Brien finished his diving career as a United States national champion and pursued a career as a swimming and diving coach. Dr. O'Brien taught swimming, diving, lifesaving, and scuba diving at the University of Minnesota and The Ohio State University for 15 years.

Dr. O'Brien's coaching accomplishments are unequaled in the sport of diving, having been United States Olympic Team coach 8 times and coach of the year 14 times. In addition, he has produced 12 Olympic medallists (5 gold) and 134 U.S. national champions, and has captured 87 U.S. National Team Championships. Dr. O'Brien has published two books, over 100 articles, and several research studies. Currently, Dr. O'Brien conducts clinics throughout the country and serves as a consultant for several organizations.

Acknowledgments

EDITORIAL BOARD

- **Charles Batterman, M.A.**—Former swimming and diving coach, MIT, Cambridge, Massachusetts; national diving champion; and author of *The Techniques of Springboard Diving*
- **Milton Costello, P.E.**—Professional engineer; pool consultant to schools, colleges, and municipalities; engineer for University of Texas and University of Illinois
- **Adolph Kiefer**—Olympic gold medal winner. Manufacturer of swimming pool equipment, Zion, Illinois
- **Arthur Mittelstaedt, Jr., Ed.D.**—Waterfront, pool, and park planner; president, Recreation Safety Institute, Ronkonkoma, New York; and professional recreation educator and landscape architect
- **Eric Mood, M.P.H.**—Former director, Department of Environmental Health, Division of Occupational and Environmental Health, Yale University, School of Medicine
- **Charles E. Pound, M.A.**—Former commissioner, Westchester County Department of Parks, Recreation and Conservation; former chairman, New York State Governor's Advisory Commission on Youth Camp Safety
- **Gaston Raffelli, P.E.**—Professional engineer and consulting pool engineer, Princeton, New Jersey
- **L. Stanley Shulman, M.A.**—Instructor of swimming and diving for over 40 years; Red Cross WSI; taught thousands of adults and children to swim and dive; consultant on diving and drowning sport-related injuries
- **Kim W. Tyson**—Aquatic coordinator, Department of Kinesiology and Health Education, University of Texas at Austin

OTHERS

- **Ken Stern**—Videographer and research assistant
- **Mike Sprain**—Research assistant
- **Mary Teslow**—Manuscript preparation

Contents

Chapter 5   Aboveground Pool Diving Accidents

Chapter 6   Inground Pool Diving Accidents

Chapter 7   Springboard/Jumpboard Diving Accidents

Chapter 9   Diving Accidents Occurring in the Natural Environment

1 The Problem in Swimming Pools and at Beaches

Thirty years ago Lawrence Rockefeller headed a Congressional Commission known as the Outdoor Recreation Resources Review Commission. Among the conclusions the Commission came to was that water would be the focal point of the recreational pursuits of Americans by the year 1980. The Commission was right about the popularity of aquatics, but it missed the target by about 10 years. Participation in aquatic activities became the number-one recreation activity of Americans in the mid-1970s. Today, it is estimated that 140 million Americans go swimming at least once each year, with many taking a dip more often.

WHERE ARE THEY SWIMMING NOW?

Fifty years ago swimming was done at the nearest lake, pond, river, or ocean beach. That has changed with the advent of the inexpensive backyard swimming pool. About half of the people who swim today do so in swimming pools. Yet, in examining the drowning statistics, only 8% of the 6000 to 7000 annual drownings occur in swimming pools. The conclusion one comes to is that pools really are the safest place to swim.

DEFINITION OF DIVING

Diving is interpreted to mean all forms of headfirst entries into water, with or without hands and arms in the front, from fixtures and equipment from which dives can be made. Equipment includes springboards, jumpboards, fixed platforms, pool decks, water slides, and starting blocks. Structures adjacent to water or extending into it from which dives can be made include piers, boats, bridges, cliffs, and so forth.

INCIDENCE OF DIVING INJURIES

In 1989, the U.S. Consumer Product Safety Commission (CPSC) summarized the diving problem in the United States as follows:

> Approximately 700 spinal cord diving injuries are estimated to occur in the U.S. annually as a result of recreational diving into residential pools, public pools and other bodies of water. It has been further estimated that there are 150,000–175,000 people presently living in the U.S. who have suffered traumatic spinal cord injury and that diving may account for 9–10% of them. The mean life expectancy for spinal cord injury victims is estimated at 30.2 years. Diving injuries are characterized by a high percentage of complete quadriplegics. Although there has been no large scale study of diving deaths, one study reports 2,700 diving related deaths during 1980–1981, another study reports that 38% of diving injuries admitted to a group of California hospitals were dead on arrival, and two additional studies showed that 10–11% of the victims died during hospitalization following a diving accident.

Victims of diving accidents resulting in spinal cord injuries are a particularly serious concern because they are a severely disabled group (wheelchair cases) who suffer for many years and require a long and very costly treatment. The typical victim who survives is a teenager or young adult who will require a lifetime of special medical treatment. Preliminary information, based on jury verdicts, indicates the estimated annual cost of these injuries could total $1.4–3.5 billion.

Spinal cord injuries (SCI) from all types of sports represent 14.2% of the annual total SCI's (7,900 total survivors) according to the University of Alabama at Birmingham. Recreational diving is estimated at 66% of 14.2% (9.37%), which is nearly twice as much as all other sports combined including football, surfing, gymnastics, skiing, trampoline, horseback riding, etc. Some of the recreational diving victims are being injured in residential and public swimming pools. This occurs when swimmers dive into shallow water from the pool deck or dive from diving boards and hit the bottom or sides of the swimming pool.

The National Swimming Pool Foundation states that nine out of ten diving injuries occur in six feet of water or less. Approximately half of the diving injuries occur in rivers, lakes and oceans according to John S. Young, M.S., et al. Good Samaritan Medical Center, Phoenix, Arizona who has studied and reported statistics on paralyzed victims. According to U.S. Diving Association personnel, there has not been an SCI injury in competitive diving in U.S. Diving Association sanctioned swimming pools.[1]

GROWING POPULARITY OF SWIMMING POOLS

The growth of swimming pools in the United States since World War II has been nothing short of phenomenal. From an estimated 10,000 pools in 1945, the country reached the 8 million figure by 2000. Before 1945, pools in the United States were mostly located in schools, colleges, Ys, Boys' Clubs, private clubs, and public agencies (cities, counties, and states); and at the homes of the rich.

Today, over 80% of pools are found in the backyards of homes; and at motels, hotels, and apartment complexes, as amenities. Advanced technology has reduced the cost of pools so that families with modest incomes are able to afford a pool. All that is needed is a backyard. For example, in the 1950s, an aboveground pool could be purchased for as little as $350. By forsaking a summer vacation for 1 year, most families with backyards could afford a pool.

Pool manufacturers and builders advertised "Why go on vacation? Create your own vacation spot in your backyard!" Inground poured concrete or gunite pools remain three to four times as costly as those that employ a sheet of vinyl as the water container. These vinyl-liner inground pools became known as "package pools." They are manufactured products that are assembled and installed by a local installer who is usually provided by the retailer.

In the first 11 years after World War II, the swimming pool industry was unregulated except for public pools, which came under state control. Then in 1956, the National Swimming Pool Institute (NSPI) was formed; in 1958, it issued its first standard, which applied only to public and semipublic pools, and was intended as guidance for their members.[2] In 1983, NSPI changed its name to the National Spa and Pool Institute.

Unfortunately, the first NSPI standard reflected more what pool manufacturers and builders were doing at that time than what they should have been doing. Standards were not based on scientific data produced through research, but instead represented a consensus of a committee composed mostly of pool builders. As we enter the next century, the NSPI standards have never realistically addressed the problem of diving safety or recommended steps needed to prevent diving injuries.

Today, more people swim in pools than at ocean and lake beaches. Home pools have been a tremendous boon to family living. There is little doubt that the annual drowning rate in this country has been reduced because of the number of children who learned to swim in backyard pools. Yet this increase in the number and use of pools has not been without its own toll. In 1977, the National Safety Council estimated that between 600 and 700 people, mostly children, drown in pools each year.[3]

According to the 1980 statistics compiled by the National Electronic Injury Surveillance System (NEISS), an estimated 112,854 were injured in pool-related accidents.[4] Although the NEISS data do not indicate the specific nature of the pool-related injuries, all were serious enough that the victim had to be taken to the emergency room of a nearby hospital. It is obvious that more data and studies are necessary on this increasing crisis of unintentional injury occurring from diving.

WHY DO PEOPLE GET HURT FROM DIVING?

The unique characteristic of diving is that people lead with their heads. Consequently, the only protection the diver has is derived from the hands and arms, which in a properly executed dive should be in front of the head and locked against the ears. On entry into the water it is essential that there be a sufficient volume of water to provide the diver with time to alter his trajectory to avoid hitting the bottom. When the water is not deep enough, the diver may not have time to change his underwater trajectory unless he is aware of the depth before he dives. For example, if the water is 3 ft deep and the diver enters at a 45 degree angle, contact with the bottom occurs within 0.3 to 0.4 of a second.

Injury to the spine may occur when the body is traveling at a modest speed. The neck (cervical region of the spine) is very flexible; and when the diver's head impacts the bottom, the injury the diver sustains (flexion, extension, compression, subluxation, or a combination) depends on the angle of the head as it strikes the bottom. The heavier the diver, the greater the force applied to the neck as the head makes contact. Making every effort to educate people about the proper technique of safe diving and the dangers associated with diving into shallow water, and preventing people from diving into water that is too shallow are essential to the prevention of these injuries. A depth of 5 ft is considered minimum by many people when diving from the deck of the pool or from any other structure no more than 12 in. above the water. See Chapters 10 and 11 for the discussion of the physics of diving and biomechanical analysis of spinal cord injuries from diving, and Chapter 15, The Dilemma.

WHO IS RESPONSIBLE?

Who is responsible for these accidents? Some say the diver did a stupid thing, or that he was horsing around and showing off. The evidence contained in this book is contrary to this notion. However, it can be concluded that the diver made a bad judgment concerning the conditions that existed where the dive was made. Responsibility involves anyone associated with the planning, design, and operation of the facility where the injury occurred, and the regulatory agencies charged with responsibility to govern these facilities (see Chapter 13).

For years, the American Red Cross (ARC) has warned people that they should familiarize themselves with the area where they intend to dive. However, such warnings imply knowledge about the nature of the bottom, the depth of the water in which the dive is to be made, and the bottom contour. Unfortunately, not everyone adequately "gets the word" or appreciates its significance. Persons assume that if a pool or a lake possesses a diving board, then it must be safe to dive into; this is a common, but specious reason in far too many situations.

Aquatic professionals must recognize that they bear the mantle of leadership in formulating a solution to the problem of head and neck injuries resulting from diving. Existing aquatic and governmental agencies and the swimming pool industry as presently constituted are either unable or unwilling to act.

Only through the combined action and effort of all aquatic professionals can the public be uniformly and properly educated about safe diving. Governmental agencies must regulate wisely; aquatics agencies must educate their members and the public; and the swimming pool industry must make a greater effort to promote a safer environment in and around swimming pools.

COSTS OF QUADRIPLEGIA

The projected cost for lifetime medical and attendant care of one quadriplegic, based on 1999 estimates computed with a very moderate inflation factor, is substantially over $2.5 million. This dollar estimate does not include the loss of earning power for that individual or the discomfort, pain, suffering, and loss of enjoyment of much of what life has to offer. If injury estimates are accurate, we are confronting medical care costs of extraordinary proportions that are increasing each year, easily in excess of a billion dollars annually. These are costs that ultimately are borne by society and its taxpayers. The societal costs are even greater if the cost of litigation, psychological services, and public social services are added; and by any estimation, these are not the outside parameters. This discussion does not fully incorporate the essence of a caring and humane society that has no dollar equivalent. There can be no real compensation for the anguish of the victim and the family, and the loss of human potential.

EARLY STUDIES OF THE PROBLEM

The diving injury mechanism was among the earliest studies in this area. In 1962, Schneider et al.[5] analyzed the spinal injuries occurring to cliff divers in Acapulco. Snyder reported on free falls, including jumps and dives from the Golden Gate Bridge in San Francisco.[6]

The problem of spinal cord injuries from unregulated diving was first documented by Rado,[7] a neurosurgeon. In 1967, he summarized a 4-year study of neck fractures resulting from diving accidents occurring in New Jersey. He concluded, "Eighty cases in 4 years becomes a frightening statistic when we realize that 54 are permanently and totally incapacitated. If this is so in New Jersey, a projection of the data across the United States would indicate conservatively that at least 500 injuries occur annually and at least 350 can be expected to be quadriplegic, a figure six times higher than the total number of paralytic polio cases in 1965."

The frequency of injury has generated substantial information on the locus where the spinal cord injury from diving may occur. For example, in 1970, Wiley[8] reported on a 6-year study of cervical spine injuries caused by diving. The 22 cases he described involved all males, with an age range from 14 to 57, and from one hospital. Of the 9 accidents occurring in swimming pools, 5 were inground and 4 were aboveground; and the other 13 occurred in lakes, streams, quarries, or surf. Wiley indicated that in the pool accidents, the water depths where the victim struck the bottom ranged from $3\frac{1}{4}$ to $5\frac{1}{2}$ ft. In the lakes and quarries, the depth ranged from $\frac{1}{2}$ to 7 ft.

In its 1974 report, the New England Spinal Cord Injury Foundation indicated that there were 18 spinal cord injuries resulting from diving in a 12-month period, with 11 occurring in the state of Massachusetts.[9] The fact that the summer season is so short in this locale makes these figures even more alarming.

By 1976, in its discussion of the problem of swimming pool injuries, the Consumer Product Safety Commission (CPSC) stated that "one of the major accident patterns associated with swimming pools was striking the bottom or sides of the pool because of insufficient depth for diving or sliding." They further indicated that "in addition to striking the bottom of the pool, people are injured when they hit protruding water pipes, ladders, or other objects in the pool."[10]

Based on further data gathered through the NEISS, the CPSC estimated in 1977 that each year between 8000 and 9000 injuries related to diving boards were sufficiently serious to require treatment at hospital emergency rooms.[11] The same source projected an annual rate of 1800 injuries related to water slides. While the number of people injured by diving from decks of pools is not isolated in this statistical accounting, we infer its inclusion in the 42,000 other injuries related to swimming pool use, as reported in the *NEISS News*.

In 1977, Kewalramani and Kraus[12] reported on 33 spinal cord injuries from diving that occurred in 1970 and 1971. Males sustained 28 injuries and females, 5. Of the total, 9 occurred in swimming pools, 15 in rivers and creeks, 6 in lakes, and 3 in the ocean.

TABLE 1.1
Sport Activity Causing Cervical Spinal
Cord Damage in 152 Individuals

Activity	Number
Diving	82
Football	16
Gymnastics	5
Snow skiing	5
Surfing	29
Track and field	3
Trampoline	2
Water skiing	7
Wrestling	3

In 1978, Shield et al.[13] of Los Angeles analyzed 10 years of data relative to cervical spinal cord injury cases caused by sports participation that were treated at the Rancho Los Amigos Hospital. As Table 1.1 indicates, diving caused 82 (53.9%) of the injuries. When surfing and water skiing injuries are added to diving, total aquatic injuries then totaled 118 (77.6%) of the spinal cord injuries reported. It is most significant to note that the number (82) of spinal cord injuries resulting from diving exceeded the total injuries (70) produced from all other sports combined.

In 1979, a very important study was reported by McElhaney et al.,[14] who made detailed analyses of neck tolerances and neck injury mechanisms. The authors developed a mathematical model to allow the prediction of the trajectory and velocity of the subjects prior to their injuries. Critical information on dangerous impact velocities was obtained through a comparison of the real accident and the simulation. Further discussion of the mechanics of diving is presented in Chapter 10.

Another data source that has provided insight into the diving problems is the National Spinal Cord Injury Data Research Center (NSCIDRC) located at Good Samaritan Hospital in Phoenix, Arizona. In 1980, this organization published a breakdown of spinal cord injuries sustained among 21 different activity categories[15] (see Table 1.2).

Table 1.2 indicates that diving injuries ranked fourth behind auto accidents, falls, and gunshot wounds as the contributor to spinal cord injuries. NSCIDRC has estimated that there are over 8000 traumatic spinal cord injuries occurring each year in the United States. Because diving represents 10.6%, it means that there are approximately 800 injuries annually resulting from people diving into some body of water. The precise number that were pool related is not known at this time. However, the estimate is that between 150 and 250 occur in swimming pools each year.

In 1986, the University of Alabama Spinal Cord Injury Care System, which is the predecessor of the Phoenix Group, published the book *Spinal Cord Injury: The Facts and Figures*.[16]

Again, particular interest in this report is Table 1.3 titled "Distribution of Sports-Related Accidents." It indicates that diving was by far the major cause of spinal cord injuries resulting from participation in sports.

In 1997, DeVivo and Sekar[17] reported a study of "Prevention of Spinal Cord Injuries that Occur in Swimming Pools. The study was supported by the National Swimming Pool Foundation (NSPF) and by grants from the National Institute on Disability and Rehabilitation Research, U.S. Department of Education, Washington, D.C. The survey of 196 persons who were injured by diving into swimming pools was conducted by telephone with the injured persons. It was interesting to note that the results in many cases were similar to the findings reported in this book. See Chapter 3 for reference to other studies that led to the writing of this publication.

TABLE 1.2
Etiology of Traumatic Spinal Cord Injury

Category	Number Reported	Cases Percent
Auto accident	842	36.5
Fall	365	15.8
Gunshot wound	268	11.6
Diving	243	10.6
Motorcycle accident	143	6.2
Hit by falling/flying object	124	5.4
Other	61	2.7
Other sports	60	2.6
Football	29	1.3
Pedestrian	29	1.2
Medical/surgical complication	28	1.2
Bicycle	22	1.0
Other vehicle	19	0.8
Fixed-wing aircraft	19	0.8
Trampoline	15	0.7
Stabbing	9	0.4
Rotating-wing aircraft	7	0.3
Snow skiing	6	0.3
Snowmobile	5	0.3
Unknown	4	0.1
Boat	2	0.1

TABLE 1.3
Distribution of Sports-Related Accidents

Activity	Number
Diving	66.0
Football	6.1
Snow skiing	3.8
Surfing	3.1
Trampoline	2.8
Other winter sports	2.3
Wrestling	2.3
Gymnastics	2.2
Horseback riding	2.0
Other	9.8

SUMMARY

It is clear that a problem exists when one considers not only the number of diving injuries but also the devastating and catastrophic nature of these injuries. The medical costs associated with a single such injury can bankrupt an individual, institution, or company. If we add to these calamities the number of deaths from drowning each year, it is understandable that some consider aquatics as a dangerous activity. The chapters that follow present the results of the most comprehensive study yet undertaken on spinal cord injuries resulting from diving. It is hoped that widespread access to this information by the public will cause people to make diving safer.

REFERENCES

1. CPSC RFP: CPSC-P-89-2061. Evaluation of Recreational Diving in Residential Swimming Pools. August 4, 1989.
2. National Swimming Pool Standards for Public and Semi-Public Pools. NSPI, 1958.
3. National Safety Council, Accident Facts, 1977.
4. NEISS Report, Consumer Product Safety Commission, March 1977.
5. Schneider et al., The effect of change in recurrent spinal trauma in high diving, *J. Bone Joint Surg.,* 44-A, 1962.
6. Survival of High-Velocity Free-Fall in Water, Civil Aeromedical Research Institute, Report 65-12, April 1965.
7. RADO, How to handle an injured diver, *Swimming Pool Data and Reference Annual* 34, 1967.
8. Wiley, J. J., Cervical Spine Injuries in Diving Accidents, University Ottawa, 1970.
9. Spinal Cord Injury Registry Report, New England Spinal Cord Injury Foundation, No 4, 1974.
10. Fact Sheet No. 8, Swimming Pools, Consumer Product Safety Commission, July 1976.
11. NEISS Report, Consumer Product Safety Commission, 1977.
12. Shield, Fox, and Stauffer, Cervical cord injury in sports, *Physician Sports Med.,* September 1978.
13. Kewalramani, L. S. and Kraus, J. F., Acute spinal cord lesion from diving: epidemiological and clinical features, *West. J. Med.,* 126: 353–361, 1977.
14. McElhaney, J. A. and Gabrielsen, M. A., Biomechanical analysis of swimming pool neck injuries, *Soc. Automotive Eng.,* 1979.
15. The Etiology of Traumatic Spinal Cord Injury. The National Spinal Cord Data Research Center (NSCIDRC) 1980.
16. DeVivo, M. J., *Spinal Cord Injury: The Facts and Figures*, University of Alabama at Birmingham, AL, 1986.
17. DeVivo, M. J. and Sekar, P., Prevention of spinal cord injuries that occur in swimming pools, *Spinal Cord,* 35, 509, 1997.

2 Laws, Regulations, and Professional Standards for Swimming Pools and Beaches

INTRODUCTION

This chapter reviews the past and present laws, regulations, and professional standards that have application to swimming pools and beaches. Readers must realize that these standards and regulations are constantly changing; therefore, determination of applicable standards is best accomplished by contacting the agency for up-to-date copies of their regulations, codes, or standards.

POOL STANDARDS, LAWS, AND REGULATIONS

FEDERAL GOVERNMENT

Agencies of the federal government have done little to establish a safe diving envelope for swimming pools or safe water depth for diving into bodies of water found in the natural environment.

U.S. Consumer Product Safety Commission

The federal agency with the primary authority to act on behalf of the consumer with respect to pool design and operation is the Consumer Product Safety Commission (CPSC), which was established by Congress in 1972. In 1976, the commission published a standard that dealt with the design and installation of water slides in swimming pools.[1] In 1985, the CPSC and the National Spa and Pool Institute (NSPI) cosponsored a national conference on swimming pool safety.[2] These groups have also conducted regional meetings on the topics of pool drownings and diving injuries. In 1988, the CPSC developed a proposed ordinance for swimming pool barriers. In 1989, the organization recommended a model ordinance for regulating swimming pool covers. In addition, the CPSC has sponsored studies about diving and effectiveness of swimming pool warning signs and labels.

Federal Housing Administration

The Federal Housing Administration (FHA) published a document in 1966 titled "Minimum Property Standards for Swimming Pools."[3] These standards applied only "to the design and construction of semiprivate swimming pools and wading pools for multifamily housing projects" that came under FHA financing.

U.S. Department of Housing and Urban Development

In 1972, the Department of Housing and Urban Development (HUD) published a booklet on home safety that contained a section on swimming pools.[4] HUD points out that "diving boards installed incorrectly or in undersized pools always present the possibility of an injury."

Department of Health and Human Services

In June of 1976, the Environmental Health Services Division of the Department of Health and Human Services (HHS, then the Department of Health, Education, and Welfare) published a pamphlet titled "Swimming Pools: Safety and Disease Control through Proper Design and Operation,"[5] which has a short section that addresses the problem of diving boards. In July of 1981, the same agency published the first guidelines for design, construction, and operation of water slide flumes.[6] These are large slides usually found at water theme parks. Some are as long as 600 ft. These guidelines have done much to reduce the number of injuries occurring in connection with the design, installation, and use of these slides. The same year the agency also published guidelines for public spas and hot tubs.[7] The only other pool standards or manuals published by federal agencies are those distributed by the various branches of the military to their bases, the National Park Service, Army Corps of Engineers, and other agencies as applicable to their properties.

STATE AND LOCAL GOVERNMENTS

The state public health departments have the jurisdiction over public swimming pools in their states. Most have issued codes, rules, and regulations covering both public and semipublic swimming pools, but have not issued regulations governing residential pools. Because most states issue their regulations for pools through their health departments, major emphasis was placed on the sanitary aspects of pools with only minimum attention to safety. Nevertheless, the regulations present the minimum legal requirements that should be known and conformed to by all designers and builders of pools within the respective state jurisdictions. Even though the states are not directly concerned with residential pools, most major cities and counties have some type of local ordinance or building code that establishes certain controls over residential pools. Rarely do these regulations relate to diving areas or diving equipment. Most ordinances deal with the need for a permit to build a pool, locating a pool on property, and erecting required fencing.

SWIMMING POOL INDUSTRY

Standards promulgated by the swimming pool industry first appeared in 1958, shortly after the establishment of the National Swimming Pool Institute (NSPI)—an industry trade association. As of 1998, the standards published by NSPI were

- ANSI/NSPI-1 1991 Standard for Public Swimming Pools
- ANSI/NSPI-2 1992 Standard for Public Spas
- ANSI/NSPI-3 1992 Standard for Permanently Installed Residential Spas
- ANSI/NSPI-4 1992 Standard for Aboveground/Onground Residential Swimming Pools
- ANSI/NSPI-5 1995 Standard for Residential Inground Swimming Pools
- ANSI/NSPI-6 1992 Standard for Residential Portable Spas
- NSPI-7 1996 Workmanship Standards for Swimming Pools and Spas
- ANSI/NSPI-8 1996 Model Barrier Code for Residential Swimming Pools, Spas, and Hot Tubs
- BSR/NSPI/WWA-9 Public Pools in Recreation Facilities

- BSR/NSPI-10 Standard for Public Swimming Spas
- BSR/NSPI-11 Standard for Residential Swim Spas

The National Spa and Pool Foundation (NSPF) has produced and disseminated the following documents:

- The Sensible Way to Enjoy Your Pool, 1983, an essential safety guide, mandatory reading
- The Sensible Way to Enjoy Your Spa or Hot Tub, 1983
- Knowing How to Dive Can Be Worth More Than Gold—It Can Be Worth Your Life
- Knowing How to Dive Is as Important as Learning How to Swim
- "Learning to Dive," a 1986 16-mm film featuring Greg Louganis, the Olympic diving champion

PROFESSIONAL ORGANIZATIONS AND VOLUNTARY AGENCIES

A number of professional groups, some with only a general interest in aquatics and others with a very specific interest, have produced publications that in one way or another address the question of safe diving conditions along with recommendations for the dimensions in the diving portion of pools. These include the National Water Safety Congress; the National Safety Council; the American Red Cross (ARC); the Recreation Safety Institute; the National Recreation and Park Association; and the American Alliance for Health, Physical Education, Recreation, and Dance (AAHPERD). The swimming pool industry publications *Pool and Spa News* and *Swimming Pool Age* have done a good job of keeping the pool industry members alert as to what is happening. Without question, one of the best programs designed to improve safety was designed by Ellis and Associates. This program has been used to train 90% of the lifeguards employed by water theme parks and, as a result, has saved many lives.

GOVERNING BODIES FOR COMPETITIVE SWIMMING AND DIVING

Groups such as United States Swimming (USS), United States Diving (USD), National Collegiate Athletic Association (NCAA), International Swim and Dive Federation (FINA), and National Federation of State High School Athletic Associations (NFSHSAA) all publish detailed specifications governing pool dimensions and equipment used in swimming and diving competition. In 1988, USD published "Dive Safety, A Position Paper" that stated in its introduction: "In 80 years of competitive diving in the United States, there has been no record of a fatality or a catastrophic injury connected with a supervised training session or diving competition." This statement refers to pools that met USD standards.

A serious mistake that the ruling bodies for competitive swimming made in the 1960s was permitting starting blocks to be placed at the shallow end of the pool. This rule was changed in 1992, but not until 50 quadriplegics had been produced by swimmers diving off starting blocks into $3\frac{1}{2}$ to 4 ft of water. See Chapter 8 for details.

COUNCIL FOR NATIONAL COOPERATION IN AQUATICS

The Council for National Cooperation in Aquatics (CNCA) published the most comprehensive resource book on the planning, design, and operation of swimming pools in this country, titled *Swimming Pools: A Guide to their Planning, Design, and Operation*, which was edited by Gabrielsen.[8] The fourth edition (1987) of the book contains specific recommendations concerning springboards, jumpboards, minitrampolines, water slides, and starting blocks. The CNCA has now been super-seded by the National Aquatic Coalition, which is now getting poised to stress aquatic safety.

AMERICAN PUBLIC HEALTH ASSOCIATION

The American Public Health Association (APHA) first published its suggested ordinances for swimming pools in the mid-1920s. Their current editions are

- Suggested Ordinances and Regulations Covering Residential Swimming Pools, 1970
- Suggested Ordinances and Regulations Covering Public Swimming Pools, 1980

The APHA has been in the forefront in attempting to establish swimming pool standards. Many states have patterned their pool state regulations after the recommendations contained in APHA publications.

NATIONAL SANITATION FOUNDATION

The National Sanitation Foundation (NSF) publishes standards related to pool pumps, filter systems, piping, valves, and fittings associated with the hydraulic system of pools, including skimmers. The organization also recommends testing conditions, procedures, and standards for chemical feeding equipment. In addition, it operates a laboratory where newly developed equipment is tested. Much of the work is published and then used by the NSPI.

AMERICAN RED CROSS

The American Red Cross (ARC), through its various publications on water safety, has been safety oriented since Commodore Longfellow started the Life Saving Service in 1914. Without question, the ARC with its training of millions of lifeguards has saved a significant number of people from drowning and also has prevented many diving accidents. The textbook *American Red Cross Lifeguarding*[9] is used as part of the training of over 250,000 lifeguards each year. Then in 1988, the ARC published the book *Emergency Water Safety*;[10] in 1992, Mosby Lifeline published for the ARC the book titled *Swimming and Diving*,[11] which contains an excellent chapter on diving safety.

OTHER VOLUNTARY GROUPS

Other voluntary groups such as the national Boy Scouts of America, Girl Scouts of the USA, YMCA, YWCA, Boys' and Girls' Clubs, and National Jewish Welfare Board have all dealt with the subject of safety in diving. They developed guidelines for minimum dimensions for diving facilities and equipment, essentially for the guidance of their constituents.

INLAND AND OCEAN BEACH STANDARDS

Few states have any laws or regulations pertaining to the operation of public swimming beaches. However, most have developed manuals for the operation of beaches that are under their jurisdiction. Missing are regulations of any kind pertaining to design of beaches operated by resort hotels, cities, and counties, as well as owners of vacation homes located on lakes or oceans. The AAHPERD and Athletic Institute published a chapter on planning bathing beaches and waterfronts.

There are, however, several agencies and organizations that have developed standards or guidelines for the management of lake and ocean beaches. They are U.S. Life Saving Association 1994—Open Water;[12] Safety Standards for the Planning, Design, Operation, and Maintenance of Inland Water Swimming Beaches[13] by the National Water Safety Congress, 1982; and Recommended Standards for Bathing Beaches by Great Lakes—Upper Mississippi River Board of State Sanitary Engineers, 1975.[14]

REFERENCES

1. Swimming Pool Slides: Safety Standards, U.S. Consumer Product Safety Commission, 1976, revised 1984.
2. National Pool and Spa Safety Conference Report, May 14, 1985, USCPSC and NSPI cosponsored the conference.
3. Minimum Property Standards for Swimming Pools, U.S. Federal Housing Authority (FHA), U.S. Government Printing Office, Washington, D.C., 1966.
4. A Design Guide for Home Safety, Department of Housing and Urban Development, prepared by Teledyne Brown Engineering, 1972.
5. Swimming Pools: Safety and Disease Control through Proper Design and Operation, U.S. Department of Health, Education, and Welfare (CDC), Atlanta, GA, 1976.
6. Suggested Health and Safety Guidelines for Recreational Water Slide Flumes, U.S. Department of Health and Human Services (CDC), Atlanta, GA, 1981.
7. Suggested Health and Safety Guidelines for Public Spas and Hot Tubs, U.S. Department of Health and Human Services (CDC), Atlanta, GA, April 1981.
8. Gabrielsen, M., Ed., *Swimming Pools: A Guide to their Planning, Design, and Operation,* Council for National Cooperation in Aquatics, Human Kinetics, Champaign, ILL, 1969, (revised in 1972, 1975, and 1986).
9. American Red Cross, *American Red Cross Lifeguarding,* Washington, D.C., 1990.
10. American Red Cross, *Emergency Water Safety,* Washington, D.C., 1988.
11. American Red Cross, *Swimming and Diving,* Mosby Lifeline, 1992.
12. Life Saving and Marine Safety. U.S. Life Saving Association, 1981.
13. Safety Standards for the Planning, Design, Operation and Maintenance of Inland Water Swimming Beaches, National Water Safety Congress, 1982.
14. Recommended Standards for Bathing Beaches, Great Lakes—Upper Mississippi River Board of State Sanitary Engineers, 1975.

3 Research Methodology

INTRODUCTION

Dr. Gabrielsen started to collect data on diving injuries in the early 1970s. Since then, with the assistance of members of the Editorial Board, data has now been collected on 601 diving injuries, of which 440 were accidents occurring in swimming pools, and 161 in water areas found in the natural environment (i.e., lakes, rivers, ocean, ponds, and quarries). This data was the basis for the information contained in this publication.

Early in the investigation it was found that the most effective way to collect information on these injuries was through accidents that were in litigation, and where an expert witness had been engaged to assist the plaintiff. Because of the severity of the injury, every diving-injured person is prone to seek compensation for the injury. Thus, evidence in litigation is the most factual type of data that can be collected.

The following previous analyses of diving injuries reported by Gabrielsen were

1. Medical Analysis of Swimming Pool Injuries, a study conducted for the United States Consumer Product Safety Commission (CPSC) by the University of Miami School of Medicine and Nova University.[1] This 1976 study recorded data on 72 swimming pool diving injuries.
2. In 1984, the Council for National Cooperation in Aquatics (CNCA) published a book titled *Diving Injuries: A Critical Insight and Recommendations*, authored by Gabrielsen[2] with the assistance of 20 others serving on the Editorial Board. This work reported on 152 diving injuries, all occurring in swimming pools.
3. In 1985, Gabrielsen[3] reported on 211 pool diving injuries at the National Pool and Spa Safety Conference, cosponsored by the CPSC and the National Spa and Pool Institute (NSPI).
4. In 1990, Nova University published the book titled *Diving Injuries: The Etiology of 486 Case Studies with Recommendations for Needed Action*.[4] Of the 486 cases, 360 were pool related and 126 injuries occurred in the natural environment.

Each of the 601 diving accidents became an independent study. A four-page data form, shown in Figure 3.1, was used to record data on each swimming pool case. The data form used for accidents occurring in the natural environment is shown in Figure 3.2.

TYPICAL DATA COLLECTION SCENARIO

To help the reader understand the complexity involved in the process of collecting data related to the accidents, a typical scenario is presented with the sources and methods employed.

1. An individual is injured in an accident involving an aquatic facility (pool, lake, river, ocean, etc.) and, as a result, is hospitalized.
2. Because of the seriousness of the injury, the victim or his family employs a law firm to represent the victim and seek damages from potential defendants. At this point the victim assumes the identity of the plaintiff in the lawsuit.

FIGURE 3.1 Pool data form.

Code Number: _____

NOVA UNIVERSITY DIVE/SLIDE RESEARCH CENTER
DATA FORM FOR RECORDING
POOL-RELATED SPINAL CORD INJURIES FROM DIVING

VICTIM

Sex (M/F): _____   Age: _____   Height: _____ ft. _____ in.   Weight: _____ lb

Married (Y/N): _____   Children: (Y/N): _____   Number: _____

Accident Date: _____/_____/_____   Day: _____   Time Day: _____ am/pm

Injury Diagnosis: _____

State/City where accident occurred: _____

Corrective Lenses: Did victim wear lenses?   Yes:_____   No:_____

Swimming/Diving Instruction Victim Received During Lifetime: (one or more)

                    Self: _____   Parents:_____   Red Cross:_____

                    YMCA:_____   Club:_____   Private:_____   School:_____

                    Others (name):_____

                    Age victim learned to swim:_____ years old

                    Member of swim team: Yes:_____   No:_____

                    Diving skill on a scale of 1-10 (10 highest) _____

POOL SPECIFICATIONS

Pool Owner: Residential:_____   Apt/Condo:_____

                          Hotel/Motel:_____   Vol. Agency:_____

                          Municipal/City:_____   Municipal/County:_____

                          Commercial:_____   Private/Country Club:_____

                          High School:_____   College:_____

                          Other:_____

Pool Specifications: Dimensions:_____

Shape: Rectangular:_____   "L":_____   "T"_____

                          Round:_____   Kidney:_____

                          Oval:_____   Free-form: _____

Location: Indoor:_____   Outdoor:_____

                          In-ground:_____   Above-ground:_____

Depth of Water: Shallow end: _____ft. _____in.   Deep end: _____ft. _____ in.

Bottom Profile: Hopper:_____   Spoon:_____   Constant/Competitive:_____

                               Shallow/sloping:_____   Shallow/constant:_____

Pool Basin Finish: Poured concrete:_____   Fiberteck:_____

                               Vinyl:_____   Gunite:_____   Other:_____

Depth Markers: Yes:_____   No:_____

          Location: Interior wall:_____   Coping:_____   Deck:_____

Pool Bottom Markings: Yes:_____   No:_____

          Describe: _____

Pool Diagram: Draw a vertical plane diagram of the pool and indicate the equipment location
                               on the last page of the data form.

Pool Equipment:

          Waterslides: Number:_____   Size:_____

                               Location in pool:_____

          Springboards: Number:_____   Length:_____

                               Height above water:_____   Aluminum:_____

                               Fiberglass:_____   Wood:_____

          Jumpboards: Number:_____   Length:_____

                               Height above water:_____

                               Fiberglass:_____   Wood:_____

          Lifeline: In place at time of accident: Yes:_____   No:_____

          Lifeguard stand(s): Number:_____

                               Location(s): _____

ENVIRONMENTAL CONDITIONS

Lighting: Was lighting a factor?   Yes:_____   No:_____

                               If yes, describe:_____

          Underwater: Number:_____   Location:_____

          Pool area: Number:_____   Location:_____

          Glare: Was glare a factor?   Yes:_____   No:_____

          (from sun/lights)   If yes, describe:_____

Water clarity: Clear:_____   Turbid:_____

                               Semi-Turbid:_____

Weather: Was weather a factor?   Yes:_____   No:_____

SUPERVISION & SAFETY FEATURES

Pool Rules: Were pool rules posted?   Yes:_____   No:_____

                           More than one set?   Yes:_____   No:_____

                           If yes, give content and location:_____

                           _____

                           Were warnings against diving/sliding

                           contained in pool rules?   Yes:_____   No:_____

Warning Signs: Were warning signs posted?   Yes:_____   No:_____

                           If yes, give content and location:_____

                           _____

                           Were there any signs specifically prohibiting diving in any

                           location in the pool?   Yes:_____   No:_____

                           If yes, describe content and location:_____

                           _____

                           Did the warning relate specifically to the circumstances

                           involved in this incident?   Yes:_____   No:_____

                           Had victim been verbally warned by any person

                           prior to the injury?   Yes:_____   No:_____

Lifeguard(s):   Was there a certified lifeguard on duty:

                           Yes:_____   No:_____   If yes, number:_____

                           Was he: Paid:_____   Volunteer:_____

                           Location of each lifeguard: _____

                           _____

DESCRIPTION OF VICTIM'S ACTION AND CONDITIONS
BEFORE AND AT THE TIME OF INJURY

Location of Dive: Specify location where dive occurred:_____

                           _____

Description of Dive: Running:_____   Standing:_____

                           Springboard:_____   Jumpboard:_____

Depth of Water: Where victim impacted bottom, based on victim's and

                           witnesses' statements: _____ft. _____in.

Arm/Hand Position: At water entry:_____

Prior Visits: Number of prior visits during: Accident year:_____

                                                                Prior years:_____

Prior Dives: Dive when injury occurred: First dive:_____

                               Second Dive:_____   Three or more:_____

                               Estimated number of dives

                               made at site during   Previous visits:_____

Accident Setting: Number of people at site:__   In site area:_____

                               Witnesses: Yes:___ No:___

                               Victim household member: Yes:_____   No:_____

                               Victim homeowner's guest: Yes:_____   No:_____

                               Small, informal gathering   Yes:_____   No:_____

                               Formal party with invitations   Yes:_____   No:_____

Substance Use: Drugs on day of accident: Yes:_____   No:_____

                               If yes, type:_____   Quantity:_____

                               Alcohol on day of accident: Yes:_____   No:_____

                               Beers consumed:_____   Time span:_____

                               Other forms of alcohol:_____

                               Blood alcohol, if taken: _____   Time span:_____

Narrative Description of Dive at Time of Accident and Events Preceding Incident:

_____

_____

_____

RESCUE PROCEDURES AND ADMISSION INFORMATION

Removal of the Victim: Dragged:_____   Lifted:_____

                               Remained in water:_____   By Self:_____

                               Spine Board or rigid device   Yes:_____   No:_____

                               CPR administered   Yes:_____   No:_____

                               Rescue Squad involved   Yes:_____   No:_____

                               Description: _____

                               _____

Hospital Admission: Name of hospital where victim was first admitted:

                               _____

Injury: Any abrasion, laceration, etc. on head?

                               If, yes, describe:_____

                               _____

ATTACH DRAWINGS AND/OR PHOTOS OF POOL AND AREA

FIGURE 3.2 Non-pool data form.

Code Number: _____

Accident Type: _____

```
┌──────────────────────────────────────────────────────────────────┐
│            NOVA UNIVERSITY DIVE/SLIDE RESEARCH CENTER              │
│                   DATA FORM FOR RECORDING                          │
│       NON-POOL-RELATED SPINAL CORD INJURIES FROM DIVING           │
└──────────────────────────────────────────────────────────────────┘
```

VICTIM

Sex (M/F): _____   Age: _____   Height: _____ ft. _____ in.   Weight: _____ lb

Married (Y/N): _____   Children: (Y/N): _____   Number: _____

Accident Date: _____/_____/_____   Day: _____   Time Day: _____ am/pm

Injury Diagnosis: _____

State/City where accident occurred: _____

Corrective Lenses: Did victim wear lenses?   Yes:_____   No:_____

Swimming/Diving Instruction Victim Received During Lifetime: (one or more)

    Self:_____   Parents:_____   Red Cross:_____

    YMCA:_____   Club:_____   Private:_____   School:_____

    Others (name):_____

    Age victim learned to swim: _____ years old

    Member of swim team: Yes:_____   No:_____

    Diving skill on a scale of 1-10 (10 highest)   _____

SITE SPECIFICATIONS

Owner: Fed. Gov.:_____   Commercial:_____

    State:_____   Resort/Hotel/Motel: _____

    Municipal/County: _____   Corporation:_____

    Municipal/City: _____   Apt./Condo:_____

    Utility:_____   Partnership:_____

    Private Individual:_____   Other:_____

Area Locations: Lake: _____   Quarry:_____

    Ocean: _____   Retention Basin: _____

    River: _____   Borrow Pit: _____

    Pond: _____   Excavation: _____

Canal: _____   Ocean Embayment: _____

Description of Site: _____

                              _____

                              _____

Facility Equipment: (Check all that were located at the facility.)

    Waterslides: Number:_____   Size:_____

                              Location:_____

    Springboards: Number:_____   Length:_____

                              Height above water:_____   Aluminum:_____

                              Fiberglass:_____   Wood:_____

    Jumpboards: Number:_____   Length:_____

                              Height above water:_____

                              Fiberglass:_____   Wood:_____

    Other: Pier - Fishing: _____   Bank - River: _____

                              Pier - Swimming: _____   Bank - Quarry: _____

                                                                   Raft: _____

                              Pier - Large Boat: _____   Other: (i.e., water skiis,

                              Boat: _____   Skidoo, surfboard):

                              Boat Dock: _____   _____

    Swimming Area: Designated?   Yes:_____   No:_____

    Lifeline: In place at time of accident: Yes:_____   No:_____

    Lifeguard stands: Number:_____

                              Location(s): _____

Depth Markers: Yes:_____   No:_____

    Location: _____

Site Diagram: Draw a vertical plane diagram of the site and indicate the equipment location
                             on the last page of the data form.

ENVIRONMENTAL CONDITIONS

Lighting: Was lighting a factor?   Yes:_____   No:_____

                             If yes, describe:_____

    Site area: Number:_____   Location:_____

    Glare: (from the sun) Was glare a factor?   Yes:_____   No:_____

                             If yes, describe:_____

Water clarity: Clear:_____   Turbid:_____

                                  Semi-Turbid:_____

Weather: Was weather a factor?   Yes:_____   No:_____

SUPERVISION & SAFETY FEATURES

Facility Rules: Were rules posted?   Yes:_____   No:_____

                                  More than one set?   Yes:_____   No:_____

                                  If yes, give content and location:_____

                                  _____

                                  Were warnings against diving/sliding

                                  contained in the rules?   Yes:_____   No:_____

Warning Signs: Were warning signs posted?   Yes:_____   No:_____

                                  If yes, give content and location:_____

                                  _____

                                  Were there any signs specifically prohibiting diving in any

                                  location at the site?   Yes:_____   No:_____

                                  If yes, describe content and location:_____

                                  _____

                                  Did the warning relate specifically to the circumstances

                                  involved in this incident?   Yes:_____   No:_____

                                  Had victim been verbally warned by any person

                                  prior to the injury?   Yes:_____   No:_____

Lifeguard(s):   Was there a certified lifeguard on duty:

                                  Yes:_____   No:_____   If yes, number:_____

                                  Was he: Paid:_____   Volunteer:_____

                                  Location of each lifeguard:_____

                                  _____

DESCRIPTION OF VICTIM'S ACTION AND CONDITIONS
BEFORE AND AT THE TIME OF INJURY

Location of Dive: Specify location where dive occurred:_____

                                  _____

Description of Dive: Running:_____   Standing:_____

Springboard:_____   Other:_____

Depth of Water: Where victim impacted bottom, based on victim's and

witnesses' statements: _____ft. _____in.

Arm/Hand Position: At water entry:_____

Prior Visits: Number of prior visits during: Accident year:_____

Prior years:_____

Prior Dives: Dive when injury occurred: First dive:_____

Second Dive:_____   Three or more:_____

Accident Setting: Number of people in site:_____   Witnesses: Yes:_____ No:_____

Small, informal gathering   Yes:_____   No:_____

Formal party with invitations   Yes:_____   No:_____

Substance Abuse: Drugs on day of accident: Yes:_____   No:_____

If yes, type:_____   Quantity:_____

Alcohol on day of accident: Yes:_____   No:_____

Beers consumed:_____   Time span:_____

Other forms of alcohol:_____

Blood alcohol, if taken: _____   Time span:_____

Narrative Description of Dive at Time of Accident and Events Preceding Incident:

_____

_____

_____

RESCUE PROCEDURES AND ADMISSION INFORMATION

Removal of the Victim: Dragged:_____   Lifted:_____

Remained in water:_____   By Self:_____

Spine Board or rigid device   Yes:_____   No:_____

CPR administered   Yes:_____   No:_____

Rescue Squad involved?   Yes:_____   No:_____

Description: _____

_____

Hospital Admission: Name of hospital where victim was first admitted:

_____

Injury: Any abrasion, laceration, etc. on head?

If, yes, describe:_____

_____

ATTACH DRAWINGS AND/OR PHOTOS OF SITE AND AREA

3. The law firm then begins collecting information about the injury including:

   • Hospital medical records including emergency care, history and physical, diagnostic imaging reports, discharge summary, etc.
   • Name and location of the site of the accident
   • Police report of the accident
   • Any witness statements taken by the police
   • Newspaper and TV reports of the accident
   • Description of the victim: age, education, sex, marital status, and background
   • The victim's account of how the accident happened
   • Any laws or codes that apply to the aquatic site

4. About this time (sometimes even earlier) the law firm looks for possible experts in aquatic safety who could help them to establish the negligence of potential defendants. The firm usually requests a curriculum vitae from the potential expert and establishes a fee schedule.
5. Possible defendants in a swimming pool case are

   • Owner of the pool (home, motel/hotel, apartment/condominium, city, school, etc.)
   • Contractor who built the pool
   • Architect if one was used
   • Manager of the pool
   • Manufacturer of the pool and pool equipment (such as diving boards and stands, water slides, etc.)
   • Owner of lakes, pond, beaches, docks, and piers

6. The law firm retains the expert. The expert then provides background information on diving injuries.
7. The expert visits the accident site and determines causation.
8. During the expert's visit to the accident site, he usually:

   • Meets with the lawyer to discuss the case
   • Meets with the plaintiff, if possible
   • Takes photos at the accident site.
   • Takes measurements of the pool or facility
   • Gets copies of documents that have been produced by the plaintiff's lawyer, such as complaint, interrogatories, affidavits, any depositions that have been taken, witness statements, and any reports submitted by the defense expert witnesses

9. The expert is asked to prepare a preliminary report or affidavit indicating the negligence of the various defendants.
10. The expert is usually deposed by the defense attorney and cross-examined by the plaintiff's attorney.

11. In addition to the expert's deposition, other depositions are taken both by the defense and the plaintiff's lawyer, mostly from witnesses to the incident. These are made available to the expert.
12. At this time, invariably, a meeting with both sides participating is called to discuss a possible settlement of the case. Of the 601 cases reported in this book, about 480(80%) were settled out of court.

It usually takes a minimum of 2 years for lawyers to prepare a case for trial. The cost ranges from $20,000 to over $100,000.

SUMMARY OF DATA SOURCES

1. During the expert's visits to accident sites, the following information is obtained:

   • Photographs of the pool or facility
   • Measurements of the pool
   • Architectural drawing of the pool or facility
   • Videotape of the facility, if taken
   • Interview with the victim

2. Other documents that are made available and reviewed in the process of data collection by the investigator include:

   • Depositions of the victim and witnesses to the accident
   • Medical records, admission and discharge summaries
   • Statements and depositions of people involved in the suit
   • Other legal documents such as the complaint, interrogatories, and trial testimony
   • Standards applicable to beaches, piers, and docks
   • All laws or regulations applicable to the facility
   • National Spa and Pool Institute (NSPI) standards
   • Police and rescue squad accident reports
   • Newspaper accounts of the accident

Many documents are produced and reviewed by the expert in order to complete the data form. (See Figure 3.3 for an example of the number of documents typically involved in a case.) Once the data form is completed, it is placed in one of the following categories:

   • Diving injuries occurring in aboveground pools
   • Injuries that occurred as a result of dives into inground pools from decks and adjacent structures
   • Dives from springboards/jumpboards
   • Dives off starting blocks

The data in each of the preceding categories was then computerized, tables were developed, and they are presented in this book in the following chapters:

Chapter 4: Composite of Data for 440 Swimming Pool Diving Accidents
Chapter 5: Analysis of Data for 105 Aboveground Pool Accidents
Chapter 6: Analysis of Data for 211 Inground Pool Accidents
Chapter 7: Analysis of Data for 92 Springboard/Jumpboard Accidents

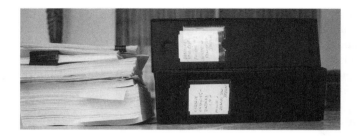

FIGURE 3.3 Example of the quantity of documents involved in a single case.

Chapter 8: Analysis of Data for 32 Starting Block Accidents
Chapter 9: Analysis of Data for 161 Accidents Occurring in the Natural Environment

REFERENCES

1. Medical Analysis of Swimming Pool Injuries, a study conducted for the United States Consumer Product Safety Commission (CPSC), University of Miami School of Medicine and Nova University, 1977.
2. Gabrielsen, M., *Diving Injuries: A Critical Insight and Recommendations,* Council for National Cooperation in Aquatics, 1984.
3. Gabrielsen, M. A., reported on 211 diving injuries at the National Pool and Spa Safety Conference, cosponsored by the U.S. Consumer Product Safety Commission (CPSC) and the National Spa and Pool Institute (NSPI), 1985.
4. Gabrielsen, M. A., *Diving Injuries: The Etiology of 486 Case Studies with Recommendations for Needed Action,* Nova University Press, Fort Lauderdale, FL, 1990.

4 Swimming Pool Diving Accidents

INTRODUCTION

This chapter records data from a total of 440 diving injuries that occurred in swimming pools. Extracted from the 440 pool-related cases are those that represent dives taken from starting blocks and springboards/jumpboards; dives and slides made from the deck and headfirst slides into inground pools; and dives made into aboveground pools. These individual analyses are presented in separate chapters, namely:

Chapter 5: Analysis of Data for 105 Aboveground Pool Accidents
Chapter 6: Analysis of Data for 211 Inground Pool Accidents
Chapter 7: Analysis of Data for 92 Springboard/Jumpboard Accidents
Chapter 8: Analysis of Data for 32 Starting Block Accidents

Combining the data from these studies yielded a total of 440 injuries. The investigators considered it essential to record the data in these four categories because of the dissimilarity of the facilities involved.

Data derived from the sources previously indicated were recorded on a four-page collection form. The data were then computerized, and various tables were developed in the following categories:

Victims
Pool facilities
Environmental factors
Pre- and postaccident events
Safety and supervision
Rescue procedures

Dives of any kind involve many elements that include human factors, techniques of diving, and environmental factors that may have influence on the dive.

VICTIMS

AGE AND SEX

As indicated in Table 4.1, of the 440 victims, 359(81.6%) were males and only 81(18.4%) were female. A surprising finding was that 15(3.4%) victims were 40 years of age or older with a mean age for males of 23.8 years and a mean age for females of 20.9 years. This is contrary to the general belief that most victims of diving injuries were teenagers.

TABLE 4.1
Age and Sex of Victims

Age	Males	Females	Total
10–12	4	6	10
13–15	38	33	71
16–18	73	10	83
19–21	70	5	75
22–24	59	6	65
25–27	36	9	45
28–30	24	4	28
31–33	20	5	25
34–36	8	1	9
37–39	13	1	14
40–42	6	1	7
43–45	2	0	2
46–48	1	0	1
49–51	1	0	1
52–54	2	0	2
55+	2	0	2
Total	359	81	440

TABLE 4.2
Height of Victims

Height (ft/in.)	Males	Females	Total
4/10	2	0	2
4/11	0	0	0
5/0	3	9	12
5/1	0	6	6
5/2	0	6	6
5/3	0	6	6
5/4	1	16	17
5/5	5	14	19
5/6	9	14	23
5/7	27	5	32
5/8	23	4	27
5/9	25	1	26
5/10	56	0	56
5/11	54	0	54
6/0	81	0	81
6/1	33	0	33
6/2	16	0	16
6/3	12	0	12
6/4	7	0	7
6/5	4	0	4
6/6	0	0	0
6/7	1	0	1
Total	359	81	440

HEIGHT AND WEIGHT

Table 4.2 gives the height of victims with 154(35.0%) of the males being 6 ft tall or taller. Table 4.3 contains the weights of the victims. The mean weight of male victims was 175 while the mean weight of females was 124.

LEVEL OF INJURY

Table 4.4 begins with the spinal cord injuries that totaled 422(95.9%). All but 18(4.1%) involved the cervical region and resulted in complete or incomplete quadriplegia. The most frequent sites were C-5 and C-5, 6, in 267(60.7%) of the cases. Where indicated in the medical record, these injuries were of the flexion type. The table continues with the 18(4.1%) injuries that did not result in paralysis. Some neurological impairment was present in 12(2.7%) of the cases, with the balance being brain hemorrhages.

SWIMMING AND DIVING INSTRUCTION

Table 4.5 indicates the age the victim learned to swim. It is very interesting to note that 405(92.0%) of the victims had learned to swim by the time they were 8 years old. Table 4.6 indicates where the victim had received his initial diving instruction. Only 80(18.2%) received any formal diving instruction. Slightly more than half (237, 53.9%) were self-taught and approximately one quarter (123, 27.9%) indicated that they had received instruction from their parents or another family member.

TABLE 4.3
Weight of Victims

Weight (lb)	Males	Females	Total
080–089	1	1	2
090–099	3	5	8
100–109	1	10	11
110–119	2	15	17
120–129	6	23	29
130–139	18	13	31
140–149	26	4	30
150–159	28	3	31
160–169	33	3	36
170–179	90	1	91
180–189	75	1	76
190–199	25	0	25
200–209	22	0	22
210–219	4	0	4
220–229	13	0	13
230–239	7	1	8
240–249	4	1	5
250–259	1	0	1
Total	359	81	440

TABLE 4.4
Level of Injury

Level	Males	Females	Total
C-1	2	1	3
C-1, 2	3	0	3
C-2	1	0	1
C-2, 3	1	0	1
C-3	1	0	1
C-3, 4	7	1	8
C-4	12	1	13
C-4, 5	50	9	59
C-5	106	23	129
C-5, 6	110	28	138
C-4, 5, 6	1	0	1
C-6	21	2	23
C-6, 7	24	8	32
C-7	3	0	3
C-7, T-1	2	0	2
T-1	1	0	1
T-1, 2	1	0	1
T-1, 2, 3	1	0	1
T-5, 6	1	0	1
T-6, 7	1	0	1
Some neurological impairment	8	4	12
Fractured jaw	0	1	1
Fractured skull	1	1	2
Fractured arm and concussion	0	1	1
Brain hemorrhage	1	1	2
Total	359	81	440

TABLE 4.5
Age Victim Learned to Swim

Age	Number
1–4	126
5–8	279
9–12	30
13 and over	5
Total	440

POOL FACILITIES

POOL OWNERSHIP

Table 4.7 identifies the owner of the property or facility where the accident occurred. Residential pools, owned and operated by individual families were involved 228(51.8%) times. Motel/hotel pools were the site of 72(16.4%) of the accidents, and apartment/condominium pools accounted for 65(14.8%) of the injuries. When these three categories of ownership were totaled, they collectively

TABLE 4.6
Source of Initial Diving Instruction

Source	Number
Self-taught	237
Parent or family member	123
City recreation department	28
American Red Cross	27
YMCA	13
School or college	12
Total	440

TABLE 4.7
Pool Ownership

Owner	Number
Residential	228
Motel/Hotel	72
Apartment/condominium	65
Municipality (city, county)	25
High school/college	24
Voluntary agency	11
Commercial	7
Private/country club	5
Others	3
Total	440

TABLE 4.8
Location

State	Number	State	Number	State	Number
Illinois	45	Colorado	8	North Carolina	2
Pennsylvania	34	Alabama	7	South Carolina	2
Florida	33	Virginia	7	Vermont	2
California	26	Kansas	6	Virgin Islands	2
Michigan	24	Missouri	6	West Virginia	2
Massachusetts	23	Tennessee	6	Alaska	1
Texas	20	Rhode Island	5	Idaho	1
Ohio	20	Georgia	4	Maine	1
New York	18	Hawaii	4	Mexico	1
New Jersey	17	Kentucky	4	Nebraska	1
Iowa	14	Maryland	4	New Hampshire	1
Indiana	13	Nevada	4	New Mexico	1
Arizona	12	Wyoming	4	Quebec, Canada	1
Minnesota	12	Oklahoma	3	South Dakota	1
Louisiana	10	Washington	3	Washington, D.C.	1
Wisconsin	10	Mississippi	2	Total	440
Connecticut	10	Montana	2		

accounted for 365(83.0%) of the accident sites. In these pools lifeguards are seldom employed to supervise pool patrons.

LOCATION BY STATE

Table 4.8 reveals that 435(98.9%) accidents occurred in 45 different states; 2(0.5%), in the Virgin Islands; and 1(0.2%) each, in Washington, D.C., Mexico, and in Canada. Illinois had the highest number of accidents at 45(10.2%) followed by Pennsylvania, California, Florida, Michigan, Massachusetts, Texas, and Ohio, all with 20(4.5%) cases or more.

POOL SHAPES

Table 4.9 identifies the shape of the pools in the four major research categories: aboveground pools (AG), inground pools (IG), inground pools with springboards (SB), and starting blocks (ST/B).

TABLE 4.9
Pool Shapes

Shape	AG	IG	SB	ST/B	Total
Conventional, rectangular	0	71	62	27	160
Circular	72	8	2	0	82
Hopper bottom	0	56	0	0	56
"L," modified "L," or lazy "L"	0	30	14	2	46
Oval	33	0	0	0	33
Kidney	0	18	10	0	28
Free form	0	14	1	0	15
"T"	0	5	3	3	11
Other shapes	0	9	0	0	9
Total	105	211	92	32	440

TABLE 4.10
Basin Composition

Finish	AG	IG	SB	ST/B	Total
Vinyl liner	105	59	43	0	207
Gunite	0	84	33	0	117
Poured concrete	0	65	16	32	113
Concrete wall/sand bottom	0	1	0	0	1
Aluminum	0	1	0	0	1
Fiberglass	0	1	0	0	1
Total	105	211	92	32	440

TABLE 4.11
Pool Markings

Marking	Yes	No	Total
Depth markings	208	232	440
Bottom markings	83	357	440
Lifeline in place	50	390	440

All the pools under the category of SB had either a hopper-bottom or spoon-shaped configuration in the deep ends.

BASIN COMPOSITION

Table 4.10 identifies the type of finish of the pool basin in the four major research categories: AG, (IG), (SB), and (ST/B). A vinyl liner was the basin finish in 207(47.0%) cases, while 230(52.3%) were either poured concrete or gunite (pneumatic concrete).

POOL MARKINGS

Table 4.11 shows the number of pools that possessed markings. Depth markers were present to aid divers in 208(47.3%) of the pools. Less common were bottom markings, found in only 83(18.9%) pools. A lifeline was in place at the time of the accident in only 50(11.4%) cases.

TABLE 4.12
Depth of Water at Impact

Depth (ft/in.)	AG	IG	SB	ST/B	Total
3/0 and under	0	79	6	0	85
3/1–3/6	105	67	1	32	205
3/7–4/0	0	39	8	0	47
4/1–4/6	0	17	18	0	35
4/7–5/0	0	6	32	0	38
5/1–5/6	0	1	13	0	14
5/7–6/0	0	1	8	0	9
6/1–6/6	0	1	4	0	5
6/7–7/0	0	0	2	0	2
Total	105	211	92	32	440

DEPTH OF WATER AT IMPACT

Table 4.12 contains the estimate of the depth of water where the victim struck the bottom or an object in the pool. Of the various points of impact, 337(76.6%) were at a depth of 4 ft or less. Because there are considerable differences among the four categories of pools, the impact depth was recorded separately for each type, that is, AG, IG, SB, and ST/B.

Readers are urged to recall that 105 victims were diving into aboveground pools that have a constant depth of $3\frac{1}{2}$ ft. Of those aboveground pools containing variable bottoms, none of the victims struck the bottom at the deepest point of the dug-out portion of the pool.

It is important to understand that the method employed to arrive at the estimated depth came from two sources: first, where the victim was spotted by other swimmers present after striking the bottom; and second, when there were eyewitnesses to the dive. Where the impact point occurred on the slope of the bottom, a range was established for both the entry point and the angle of underwater trajectory, and a mean was calculated. This was the figure that was recorded.

ENVIRONMENTAL FACTORS

CLARITY OF WATER

Table 4.13 provides data on the clarity of the pool water. It was the judgment of witnesses that in 17(3.9%) of the cases the water was turbid (cloudy), semiturbid in 67(15.2%) instances, and clear on 355(80.7%) occasions. In one case the pool was empty.

TABLE 4.13
Clarity of Water

Clarity	Number
Empty	1
Clear	355
Semiturbid	67
Turbid	17
Total	440

<table>
<tr><td colspan="4">

TABLE 4.14
Lighting and Weather

</td><td colspan="2">

TABLE 4.15
Victim: Guest or Owner

</td></tr>
</table>

Factor	Yes	No	Total		Victim	Number
Lighting	137	303	440		Guest	427
Weather	3	437	440		Owner	13
					Total	440

LIGHTING AND WEATHER

Table 4.14 presents two environmental factors, namely, lighting and weather. Lighting, that is, illumination in and around the pool, was found to be factor in 137(31.1%) of the cases. Weather was a factor in only 3(0.7%) of the accidents.

PRE- AND POSTACCIDENT EVENTS

This section covers the elements related to the pre- and postaccident events, as well as the circumstances directly related to the accident and a description of the specific activity involved.

VICTIM: GUEST OR OWNER

Table 4.15 addresses the issue of whether the victim was an owner or a guest. In 427(97.0%) cases the victims were guests or visitors. Only 13(3.0%) of the victims were members of the household, or owners or staff members of the motels/hotels or apartments/condominiums.

TIME AND DAY OF ACCIDENT

Table 4.16 summarizes the time the accidents occurred and shows that the daylight hours between 2 and 6 P.M. accounted for 208(47.3%) of the accidents. Accidents in the P.M. hours totaled 396(90.0%) while A.M. accidents were much less frequent, totaling only 44(10%). Three days—Friday, Saturday, and Sunday—accounted for 267(60.7%) of the accidents.

MONTH OF ACCIDENT

As expected, 291(66.1%) of the accidents occurred during the summer months of June, July, and August (Table 4.17), with July alone representing nearly one third (129, 29.3%) of the cases.

YEAR OF ACCIDENT

Table 4.18 records the years in which the accidents occurred.

VICTIM'S VISITS TO THE POOL

Tables 4.19 to 4.21 address the victim's familiarity with the pool. The data point out that nearly two thirds of the victims were visiting the pool for the first time, and slightly less than two thirds

TABLE 4.16
Time and Day of Accident

Time Interval	Mon.	Tue.	Wed.	Thu.	Fri.	Sat.	Sun.	Total
12:00–01:59 A.M.	3	0	0	1	4	6	6	20
02:00–03:59 A.M.	2	1	2	1	2	3	4	15
04:00–05:59 A.M.	1	0	0	0	0	0	0	1
06:00–07:59 A.M.	1	0	0	0	0	1	0	2
08:00–09:59 A.M.	0	0	0	0	0	1	1	2
10:00–11:59 A.M.	0	0	0	1	1	1	1	4
12:00–01:59 P.M.	3	5	4	5	5	6	5	33
02:00–03:59 P.M.	3	6	6	12	17	23	22	89
04:00–05:59 P.M.	11	11	14	14	26	24	19	119
06:00–07:59 P.M.	4	4	5	6	6	12	18	55
08:00–09:59 P.M.	5	4	4	7	7	11	11	49
10:00–11:59 P.M.	6	2	14	5	5	9	10	51
Total	39	33	49	52	73	97	97	440

TABLE 4.17
Month of Accident

Month	Number
January	13
February	15
March	12
April	19
May	32
June	73
July	129
August	89
September	20
October	14
November	12
December	12
Total	440

TABLE 4.18
Year of Accident

Year	Number	Year	Number
Before 1970	3	1981	33
1970	11	1982	36
1971	11	1983	40
1972	15	1984	27
1973	12	1985	22
1974	14	1986	15
1975	21	1987	19
1976	27	1988	18
1977	24	1989	14
1978	22	1990	0
1979	26	1991	2
1980	28	Total	440

TABLE 4.19
Victim's Visits to the Pool

Visits	First	Prior	Total
None	273	0	273
One or two	0	75	75
Three or more	0	92	92
Total	273	167	440

TABLE 4.20
Dives Made on Prior Visits

Dives	Number
None	68
One to three	23
Four or more	76
Total	167

were injured on their first dive. This is the most significant finding when considering which adults are at greatest risk.

Table 4.19 indicates that in 273 (62.0%) cases, the victim was visiting the pool for the first time.

TABLE 4.21
Dives Made on Day
of Accident

Dives	Number
First	270
Two or three	110
Four or more	60
Total	440

TABLE 4.22
Type of Social Setting

Setting	Number
Informal	356
Formal	84
Total	440

TABLE 4.23
Substance Abuse

Substance	Yes	No	Total
Alcohol	179	261	440
Drugs	7	433	440

DIVES MADE ON PRIOR VISITS

Of the 167(38.0%) individuals who had previously visited the accident site, 99(59.3%) had made at least one previous dive. When added to the individuals who had never been to the site previously, (273, 62.0%), a total of 341(77.5%) had never dived into the pool before the day of their accident (see Table 4.20).

DIVES MADE ON DAY OF ACCIDENT

Table 4.21 shows 270(61.4%) were injured on their first dive into the pool.

TYPE OF SOCIAL SETTING

The type of social gathering involved is indicated in Table 4.22. Only 84(19.1%) were attending a formal party where invitations had been sent. Most of these were company parties. The other 356(80.9%) were participating in a type of informal social activity, most of which were impromptu get-togethers of people ranging in number from 3 to 30.

SUBSTANCE ABUSE

As shown in Table 4.23, only 7(1.6%) victims admitted or were identified by others to have used any form of drugs on the day of their accident. On the other hand, 179(40.7%) of the victims had consumed some form of alcoholic beverage (mostly beer) within a 12-h period before the injury. According to the victims' own testimony, and those of eyewitnesses, the majority of accident victims were not intoxicated. A residential pool party was the predominant scene where alcohol was consumed.

TABLE 4.24
Posted Rules and Warning Signs

Instructions	Yes	No	Total
Posted rules	225	215	440
Warning signs	68	372	440

TABLE 4.25
Lifeguard on Duty

Lifeguard	Number
Yes	104
No	336
Total	440

TABLE 4.26
Person Making Rescue

Rescuer	Number
Friends	327
Lifeguard	74
Emergency medical services (EMS)	27
Self	9
Security guard	3
Total	440

TABLE 4.27
Use of Spineboard and CPR

Technique	Yes	No	Total
Spineboard	60	380	440
CPR	57	383	440

SAFETY AND SUPERVISION

Safety and supervision include the efforts of owners to provide instructions and warnings.

POSTED RULES AND WARNING SIGNS

Table 4.24 shows the presence of posted rules. Rules posted somewhere within the pool area regulating the action of patrons were evident at 225(51.1%) of the accident sites. Only 43(9.8%) contained a rule prohibiting diving. In only 68(15.5%) of the cases were there any signs specifically warning pool users not to dive in the vicinity where the injury, in fact, occurred.

LIFEGUARD ON DUTY

A lifeguard was on duty in only 104(23.6%) of the pools involved in these accidents, as shown in Table 4.25. These pools were invariably located in public (city or county), school, or club facilities.

RESCUE PROCEDURES

It is important to educate the public as to the proper procedures to follow when a person is suspected of having a spinal injury.

PERSON MAKING RESCUE

Table 4.26 identifies the person who made the initial rescue of the victim from the pool. The vast majority of the victims—327(74.3%)—were rescued by friends or other swimmers who were nearby. Lifeguards performed only 74(16.8%) rescues.

USE OF SPINEBOARD AND CARDIOPULMONARY RESUSCITATION

A disturbing fact is revealed in Table 4.27: in only 60(13.6%) cases was the victim removed from the water using a spineboard. This means that the vast majority were lifted, pulled, or dragged out of the water by friends who, in general, were not aware of the injury. Rescue breathing, or cardiopulmonary resuscitation (CPR), was employed in 57(13.0%) cases. This implies that the rescue of the victim was probably achieved within a minute or two from the time of injury.

SUMMARY

This chapter presents an overview, a consolidation, and a summary of the data related to all 440 diving injuries that occurred in swimming pools. As mentioned initially, the subcategories of these data are presented separately as follows:

- Chapter 5: Analysis of Data for 105 Aboveground Pool Accidents
- Chapter 6: Analysis of Data for 211 Inground Pool Accidents
- Chapter 7: Analysis of Data for 92 Springboard/Jumpboard Accidents
- Chapter 8: Analysis of Data for 32 Starting Block Accidents

These chapters contain additional details and observations concerning issues unique to each of these pool configurations.

5 Aboveground Pool Diving Accidents

INTRODUCTION

This chapter contains the findings related to injuries that occurred as a result of people diving or sliding into aboveground swimming pools. Of the 440 cases recorded in this book, 105(23.9%) occurred as a result of these dives.

The uniqueness of aboveground pools, as the term implies, is that the bottom is set on the ground rather than in the ground. By far, aboveground pools outnumber inground pools on a ratio as high as 4:1. The best estimate is that there are over 6 million aboveground pools.

The configuration of aboveground pools related to the size and shape is substantially the same, with practically all having a 4-ft wall and a water depth of **3½** ft. One variation is that some aboveground pools have what is identified as a variable-depth bottom. There is no question that the aboveground pool has been a boon to family living. It has created an important new home recreation opportunity, and there is no doubt that because of the number of children who have learned to swim in these pools, many drownings have been prevented.

Data derived from the sources previously indicated were recorded on a four-page collection form. The data were then computerized, and various tables were developed in the following categories:

- Victims
- Pool facilities
- Environmental factors
- Pre- and postaccident events
- Safety and supervision
- Rescue procedures

SOME BACKGROUND ON ABOVEGROUND POOLS

The development of aboveground swimming pools in the United States represents a phenomena of the post-World War II era. No other sport facility approaches the spectacular growth of these family-type pools, which in 1999 had reached a total of 6 million.

Initially, the attraction was the low cost and the opportunity for almost instant swimming. A qualified crew was able to erect a pool in one or two days. In addition to the low cost and short installation time, the other features that attracted customers were few local ordinances applied to these pools, a building permit was not required, and the maintenance and operation of these pools was simple.

Aboveground pools have a simple construction. The following components go into the making of the pool: the wall; the supporting structure; the vinyl liner; the seat or rim on top that locks in the liner; a ladder for access to the pool; and the pump, filter, and piping, which provide for water circulation. The company that sells the pool manufactures few, if any, of these parts. They simply repackage the necessary components.

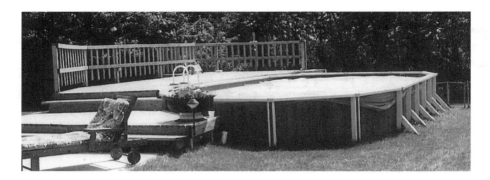

FIGURE 5.1 Typical modern aboveground pool with attached deck.

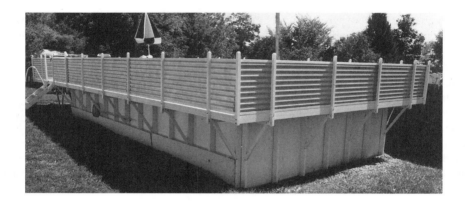

FIGURE 5.2 Fence attached to pool is a safety measure preventing people from running outside of the pool and diving over the rim of the pool.

In the 1980s, it became apparent that people wanted more than just a pool in the middle of their backyard. Today, the backyard aboveground pool resembles an inground pool, but the addition of elaborate decks, lounging areas, and other amenities has brought the cost of aboveground pools very close to that of inground vinyl-liner pools (Figures 5.1 and 5.2). As a matter of fact, inground vinyl-liner pools were the direct result of some creative engineers who, after examining the aboveground pool, said, "We can put this pool in the ground, all we need is a rigid wall to hold back the earth." Thus, the vinyl-liner inground pool was born.

The development of aboveground pools was not accomplished without its problems. The most serious was the sudden increase in the number of people who became paralyzed for life as a result of diving into aboveground pools. The exact number of quadriplegic victims is not known, but the aboveground pools of one of the major manufacturers were involved in accidents resulting in over 100 such victims.

It is estimated that over 95% of all dives into aboveground pools are performed by children. Of the 105 spinal cord injuries recorded in this chapter, no one was below 13 years of age, and 46 were over the age of 21.

At the close of the twentieth century, no federal, state, or local laws, rules, or regulations have been published to govern, for instance, the design of aboveground pools, their location on home property, and the safe operation of these pools. Only the National Spa and Pool Institute (NSPI) has developed standards for the design and operation of aboveground pools.

TABLE 5.1
Age and Sex of Victims

Ages	Males	Females	Total
10–12	0	0	0
13–15	7	6	13
16–18	12	6	18
19–21	25	3	28
22–24	10	1	11
25–27	8	2	10
28–30	7	1	8
31–33	6	1	7
34–36	3	1	4
37–39	5	0	5
40–42	1	0	1
Total	84	21	105

TABLE 5.2
Height of Victims

Height (ft/in.)	Males	Females	Total
5/0	0	3	3
5/1	0	3	3
5/2	0	0	0
5/3	0	2	2
5/4	1	4	5
5/5	1	5	6
5/6	3	1	4
5/7	6	2	8
5/8	5	1	6
5/9	4	0	4
5/10	16	0	16
5/11	17	0	17
6/0	18	0	18
6/1	5	0	5
6/2	4	0	4
6/3	3	0	3
6/4	1	0	1
Total	84	21	105

VICTIMS

AGE AND SEX

Tables 5.1 to 5.3 suggest that individuals at greatest risk are males, either adults or teenagers of adult size.

Table 5.1 indicates the following interesting factors:

- Males in the 19 to 21 years of age category represented the greatest number of victims.
- Female victims were considerably younger than were male victims.
- The age bracket from 16 to 21 represented 37(44.0%) of the 84 male victims, while 12(57.1%) of the 21 female victims were below the age of 19.
- Of particular significance is the range of age of the victims, which was from 13 to over 40.

HEIGHT AND WEIGHT

Table 5.2 indicates that 64(61.0%) of the males were 5 ft 10 in. or over while Table 5.3 indicates that 62(59.0%) weghed 170 lb or more.

LEVEL OF INJURY

Table 5.4 indicates the level of the injury to the spinal cord.

SWIMMING AND DIVING INSTRUCTION

Table 5.5 shows the age when victims learned to swim. Of the 105 victims, 100(95.2%) had learned to swim by the time they were 8 years old.

Table 5.6 reveals where the victim received instruction in how to dive. The majority were self-taught.

TABLE 5.3
Weight of Victims

Weight (lb)	Males	Females	Total
110–119	0	4	4
120–129	3	6	9
130–139	5	8	13
140–149	3	1	4
150–159	5	1	6
160–169	6	1	7
170–179	12	0	12
180–189	30	0	30
190–199	7	0	7
200–209	8	0	8
210–219	2	0	2
220–229	3	0	3
Total	84	21	105

TABLE 5.4
Level of Injury

Level	Males	Females	Total
C-1	1	0	1
C-1, 2	1	0	1
C-2	1	0	1
C-2, 3	0	0	0
C-3	1	0	1
C-3, 4	3	1	4
C-4	1	1	2
C-4, 5	15	4	19
C-5	24	6	30
C-5, 6	34	8	42
C-4, 5, 6	0	0	0
C-6	1	1	2
C-6, 7	1	0	1
T-5, 6	1	0	1
Total	84	21	105

TABLE 5.5
Age Victim Learned to Swim

Age	Number
1–4	35
5–8	65
9–12	5
13 and over	0
Total	105

TABLE 5.6
Source of Initial Diving Instruction

Source	Number
Self-taught	60
Parent or family member	30
American Red Cross	6
School or college	4
City recreation department	3
YMCA	2
Total	105

DIVING SKILL

A subjective judgment was made relative to the diving ability of the victims. It was based on review of the deposition of the victims; and testimonies of parents, spouses, or witnesses familiar with the victims' swimming and diving backgrounds. Very few victims had any formal swimming or diving training. On a scale of 1 to 10, all were rated below the 5 level with most at the 3 level.

POOL FACILITIES

POOL OWNERSHIP

All 105 of the aboveground pools were located in residential settings, as shown in Table 5.7.

LOCATION BY STATE

Table 5.8 indicates the state where the accident occurred. It is interesting to note that the majority occurred in northern states.

TABLE 5.7
Pool Ownership

Owner	Number
Residential	105
Total	105

TABLE 5.8
Location by State

State	Number	State	Number
Illinois	16	Colorado	2
Massachusetts	15	Arizona	1
Michigan	9	Florida	1
New Jersey	9	Louisiana	1
Pennsylvania	9	Montana	1
New York	8	Rhode Island	1
Connecticut	6	Tennessee	1
Ohio	6	Vermont	1
Iowa	5	Washington	1
Minnesota	4	West Virginia	1
Wisconsin	4	South Dakota	1
California	2	Total	105

POOL SHAPES AND DIMENSIONS

The variety of pools is shown in Table 5.9. More of the accidents occurred in round pools (72, 68.6%) than in oval-shaped pools (33, 31.4%). Nine of the pools had variable-depth bottoms with a maximum depth of **5½** ft.

BASIN FINISH

Table 5.10 indicates the basin finish. Every one of the pools involved in the study had a vinyl liner as the water container. An interesting fact that the study revealed was the increasing use of a "pebbled pattern" in the vinyl, reportedly for aesthetic purposes. Some of the vinyl liners were embossed while others were smooth. All were some shade of blue; none were white.

POOL MARKINGS

Of the 105 pools studied, only 5(4.8%) had any depth markers on them, as shown in Table 5.11. With respect to the placement of any type of markings on the pool bottom, none of the pools involved had any. In seven of the pools, the vinyl on the wall was a darker color as contrasted with the pool bottom.

SLIDES AND JUMPBOARDS

Five of the pools had slides. Slides in two pools were located on the deck and in the other three, on the outside placed on the ground. One pool had a 3-ft jumpboard placed on the deck.

TABLE 5.9
Pool Shapes and Dimensions

Shape and Dimensions (ft)	Number		
Round		Oval	
Size		*Size*	
12	2	12 × 24	8
15	2	14 × 24	4
18	10	14 × 27	1
20	12	15 × 30	10
21	1	16 × 30	1
24	40	15 × 31	1
25	1	16 × 32	4
26	1	18 × 33	2
27	1	18 × 36	1
28	2	15 × 40	1
		Total	105

TABLE 5.10
Basin Composition

Finish	Number
Vinyl liner	105
Gunite	0
Poured concrete	0
Concrete wall/ sand bottom	0
Aluminum	0
Fiberglass	0
Total	105

TABLE 5.11
Pool Markings

Marking	Yes	No	Total
Depth markings	5	100	105
Bottom markings	0	105	105
Lifeline in place	0	105	105

DECKS AND LADDERS

Pools had decks attached to or abutting the rim of the pool in 72 cases. Most of the decks went only partially around the pool perimeter. "A-frame" ladders provided ingress and egress from 19 of the pools.

ENVIRONMENTAL FACTORS

CLARITY OF WATER

Pools were deemed to have cloudy or semiturbid water in 24(22.8%) of the 105 cases studied according to witnesses. All other pools were reported to have water clear enough so that the bottom was visible (Table 5.12).

LIGHTING AND WEATHER

As shown in Table 5.13, in only 30(28.6%) of the accidents was lighting a factor. From the information derived from witnesses to the accident, lighting in these cases was poor to inadequate. Weather was not a significant factor in any of the 105 cases studied.

TABLE 5.12
Clarity of Water

Clarity	Number
Empty	0
Clear	81
Semiturbid	24
Turbid	0
Total	105

TABLE 5.13
Lighting and Weather

Factor	Yes	No	Total
Lighting	30	75	105
Weather	0	105	105

TABLE 5.14
Victim: Guest or Owner

Victim	Number
Guest	103
Owner	2
Total	105

TABLE 5.15
Time and Day of Accident

Time Interval	Mon.	Tue.	Wed.	Thu.	Fri.	Sat.	Sun.	Total
12:00–01:59 A.M.	0	0	0	1	1	1	1	4
02:00–03:59 A.M.	1	0	0	0	1	1	1	4
04:00–05:59 A.M.	0	0	0	0	0	0	0	0
06:00–07:59 A.M.	0	0	0	0	0	0	0	0
08:00–09:59 A.M.	0	0	0	0	0	1	1	2
10:00–11:59 A.M.	0	0	0	0	0	0	0	0
12:00–01:59 P.M.	2	3	2	2	3	2	2	16
02:00–03:59 P.M.	1	2	3	1	2	3	4	16
04:00–05:59 P.M.	3	1	4	3	2	4	3	20
06:00–07:59 P.M.	2	1	3	2	1	4	10	23
08:00–09:59 P.M.	2	1	1	1	0	3	2	10
10:00–11:59 P.M.	2	1	0	0	0	3	4	10
Total	13	9	13	10	10	22	28	105

PRE- AND POSTACCIDENT EVENTS

This section covers the elements related to the pre- and postaccident events, as well as the circumstances directly related to the accident and a description of the specific activity involved.

VICTIM: GUEST OR OWNER

As shown in Table 5.14, of the 105 accidents, 103(98.1%) of the victims were guests of the pool owners or their children. The other two (1.9%) were members of the household.

TIME AND DAY OF ACCIDENT

Table 5.15 reflects the time and day of the week that the accident occurred. Saturday and Sunday together represented 50(47.6%) of the accidents. The most frequent time period was between 4 and 8 P.M.

MONTH AND YEAR OF ACCIDENT

Table 5.16 indicates the month in which the injury to the victim occurred, and Table 5.17 records the years in which the accidents occurred. All but 16(15.2%) of the 105 accidents occurred in the three summer months: June, July, and August. Of these accidents, 90(85.7%) occurred in the time frame between 1973 and 1991.

TABLE 5.16
Month of Accident

Month	Number
January	4
February	0
March	0
April	1
May	4
June	16
July	40
August	33
September	4
October	0
November	0
December	3
Total	105

TABLE 5.17
Year of Accident

Year	Number	Year	Number
Before 1970	1	1981	6
1970	4	1982	5
1971	5	1983	2
1972	5	1984	3
1973	5	1985	4
1974	5	1986	3
1975	8	1987	5
1976	9	1988	0
1977	8	1989	1
1978	10	1990	0
1979	11	1991	0
1980	5	Total	105

VICTIM'S VISITS TO THE POOL

An important finding from this study focuses on the risk involved for first-time visitors to a backyard pool. Table 5.18 indicates that of the 105 cases studied, 70(66.7%) of the injuries occurred on the victim's first visit to the pool.

DIVES MADE ON PRIOR VISITS

Of the 35 individuals who had previously visited the pool, only 4 had made a previous dive, indicating that only 3.8% of all those injured had made a dive before the day of the accident. (Table 5.19).

DIVES MADE ON DAY OF ACCIDENT

Table 5.20 shows 73(69.5%) of the 105 victims were injured on their first dive into the pool.

TABLE 5.18
Victim's Visits to the Pool

Visits	First	Prior	Total
None	70	0	70
One or two	0	30	30
Three or more	0	5	5
Total	70	35	105

TABLE 5.19
Dives Made on Prior Visits

Dives	Number
None	31
One to three	4
Four or more	0
Total	35

TABLE 5.20
Dives Made on Day of Accident

Dives	Number
First	73
Two to three	22
Four or more	10
Total	105

TABLE 5.21
Activity Resulting in Injury

Activity	Number
Dive from the deck attached to pool	67
Standing dive from ladder attached to pool	15
Standing dives from adjacent structures (Picnic table, car roof, garage roof, roof of house, porch, porch railing, roof of porch)	7
Slide (two dives from top, four headfirst slides)	6
Running dive from outside of pool over rim	4
Cannonball from deck	2
Sailor's dive from deck	1
Standing dive from elevated 3-ft platform	1
Dive from 3-ft jumpboard located on deck	1
Thrown in pool from deck of pool	1
Total	105

ACTIVITY RESULTING IN INJURY

The activity of diving from the deck attached to or abutting the pool's rim produced 67(63.8%) of the injuries, as shown in Table 5.21. Dives made from structures located in close proximity to the pool resulted in 7(6.7%) of the injuries.

TYPE OF SOCIAL SETTING

Of the 101 accidents (96.2%), the event bringing the victim to the pool was an informal, usually spontaneous, social gathering ranging in number from 4 to over 20 people. In only four of the cases was the gathering a formal event planned in advance with verbal or written invitations (Table 5.22).

TABLE 5.22
Type of Social Setting

Setting	Number
Informal	101
Formal	4
Total	105

TABLE 5.23
Substance Abuse

Substance	Yes	No	Total
Alcohol	44	61	105
Drugs	0	105	105

TABLE 5.24
Posted Rules and Warning Signs

Instructions	Yes	No	Total
Posted Rules	4	101	105
Warning signs	12	93	105

TABLE 5.25
Lifeguard on Duty

Lifeguard	Number
Yes	0
No	105
Total	105

SUBSTANCE ABUSE

As shown in Table 5.23, 44(41.9%) of the victims indicated that they had consumed some form of alcoholic beverage (mostly beer); 11(10.5%) had consumed some other form of alcohol. Not one victim claimed to have been under the influence of drugs.

SAFETY AND SUPERVISION

The supervision of pool guests was in most instances claimed to be by one or both of the parents when youth were involved. They were usually the pool owners. No qualified person with certification by the American Red Cross (ARC) or any other agency was in charge of the swimmers.

POSTED RULES AND WARNING SIGNS

Only 12(11.4%) of the pools had any signs that warned against diving and only 4(3.8%) of the pools involved had posted rules for the use of the pool. There was considerable disagreement among witnesses as to whether anyone had warned swimmers verbally that diving was not permitted. Victims interviewed were adamant that they had not been warned by anyone (see Table 5.24).

LIFEGUARD ON DUTY

In no case did homeowners provide a lifeguard, as shown in Table 5.25.

RESCUE PROCEDURES

PERSON MAKING RESCUE

As indicated in Table 5.26, paramedics, or emergency medical services (EMS), removed only five (4.8%) of the victims from the pool.

USE OF SPINEBOARD AND CARDIOPULMONARY RESUSCITATION

Six (5.7%) victims were removed using a spineboard, as shown in Table 5.27. This means that 99(94.3%) were lifted, pulled, or dragged out of the water by friends who, in general were not

TABLE 5.26
Person Making Rescue

Rescuer	Number
Friends	100
EMS	5
Total	105

TABLE 5.27
Use of Spineboard and CPR

Technique	Yes	No	Total
Spineboard	6	99	105
CPR	15	90	105

aware that the victim had fractured his neck. Artificial resuscitation was applied in 15(14.3%) of the cases. The procedures employed involved both mouth-to-mouth and cardiopulmonary resuscitation (CPR).

CONCLUSIONS

The Editorial Board studied the data on the injuries, which occurred from dives made into aboveground swimming pools. The Board members have concluded the following as to the causes of these serious injuries:

1. The most alarming fact was that 103(98.1%) of the victims were guests of the owner of the pool or some member of the family.
2. The event that brought them to the pool was an informal get-together. Only four (3.8%) were formal events, usually one celebrating an occasion.
3. Decks and ladders were attached to the pools in 72(68.6%) of injury cases.
4. An amazing fact was that there were 20 different sizes and shapes of pools.
5. There were 12 different locations of the dives made by the victims.
6. Not a single victim was aware that he could break his neck diving into the pool.
7. There were no warning signs prohibiting diving in 93(88.6%) of the 105 pools.
8. Of the 105 injuries, 4(3.8%) were a result of the victim running outside of the pool and diving over the rim of the pool. This would not have happened if there was a fence (see Figure 5.2).
9. In 30(28.6%) of the cases, the lighting level was below standards with no underwater light illuminating the pool bottom.
10. There were five water slides, two located on the deck and three outside of the pool with the end of the slide placed over the rim of the pool.
11. It was a shock to learn that only five (4.8%) pools had any depth markers.
12. One of the pools actually had a 3-ft jumpboard on the deck. The manufacturer actually had advertised that it was available for use on decks of aboveground pools.
13. In 44(41.9%) cases the victim had consumed some form of alcoholic beverage, mostly beer.
14. First-time visitors represented 66(62.9%) of the 105 victims.
15. When the victims were interviewed, 15(14.3%) claimed that their hands struck the bottom first and slid on the vinyl liner, and the next thing they remembered was their head hitting the bottom.
16. In only 19(18.1%) of the cases was the owner of the pool present at the time of the accident.
17. Friends that were at the pool rescued 100(95.2%) of the victims. A spineboard was used in only six (5.7%) of the cases, most by EMS.
18. Of the victims, 90(85.7%) claimed that they had never been formally taught how to dive. They had taught themselves or had been instructed by a parent or family member.

6 Inground Pool Diving Accidents

INTRODUCTION

The data presented in this chapter are from 211 diving injuries that occurred as a result of people diving into inground swimming pools. Excluded from the data are those dives recorded in Chapter 5 in aboveground pools, as well as those recorded in Chapter 7 from springboards/jumpboards, and in Chapter 8 from starting blocks. It is significant to note that when the 105 aboveground pools cases and the 32 starting block cases are added to the 211 cases, the total number of shallow water dives comes to 348(79.1%) of the total 440 cases evaluated, a very significant figure.

Until 1950, all pools were of the inground type. Then came the aboveground pools, which in 1999 outnumbered inground pools by a margin of 4:1. These are practically all located in backyards of homes. (Later, in Table 6.9, a list of the pool shapes involved in this chapter is given.) Most inground pools today fall under the category of public and semipublic pools. Some motels and apartment complexes have added other recreation facilities such as fitness centers, volleyball courts, and table tennis (ping-pong) tables to their pools. A serious error occurs at some motel/hotel and apartment/condominium outdoor pools when the proprietors fail to fence the pool with self-closing and self-latching gates.

Once the data for the 211 cases were collected (see Chapter 3 on methodology) they were computerized and tables were prepared and placed under the following categories:

- Victims
- Pool facilities
- Environmental factors
- Pre- and postaccident events
- Safety and supervision
- Rescue procedures

VICTIMS

AGE AND SEX

As indicated in Table 6.1, of the 211 victims, 170(80.6%) were male and 41(19.4%) were female. With respect to the age of the victims, there was a range from 10 to 60 years with 99(46.9%) in the age range of 19 to 27. This is contrary to the general belief that most victims of diving injuries are teenagers. Single victims numbered 150(71.1%) while 61(28.9%) were married.

HEIGHT AND WEIGHT

Table 6.2 gives the height of the victims. The height of male victims was 5 ft 10 in. or more in 123(58.3%) cases, while 12(5.7%) women were 5 ft 6 in.

TABLE 6.1
Age and Sex of Victims

Ages	Males	Females	Total
10–12	4	2	6
13–15	16	16	32
16–18	26	2	28
19–21	29	2	31
22–24	34	4	38
25–27	23	7	30
28–30	11	2	13
31–33	7	4	11
34–36	2	0	2
37–39	7	1	8
40–42	3	1	4
43–45	2	0	2
46–48	1	0	1
49–51	1	0	1
52–54	2	0	2
55+	2	0	2
Total	170	41	211

TABLE 6.2
Height of Victims

Height (ft/in.)	Males	Females	Total
4/10	2	0	2
4/11	0	0	0
5/0	2	3	5
5/1	0	3	3
5/2	0	3	3
5/3	0	3	3
5/4	0	6	6
5/5	2	6	8
5/6	4	12	16
5/7	13	2	15
5/8	10	2	12
5/9	14	1	15
5/10	24	0	24
5/11	24	0	24
6/0	40	0	40
6/1	19	0	19
6/2	5	0	5
6/3	7	0	7
6/4	2	0	2
6/5	1	0	1
6/6	0	0	0
6/7	1	0	1

TABLE 6.3
Weight of Victims

Weight (lb)	Males	Females	Total
80–89	1	1	2
90–99	2	4	6
100–109	0	5	5
110–119	1	6	7
120–129	2	14	16
130–139	9	3	12
140–149	12	3	15
150–159	17	2	19
160–169	16	1	17
170–179	48	1	49
180–189	29	0	29
190–199	13	0	13
200–209	7	0	7
210–219	0	0	0
220–229	7	0	7
230–239	3	1	4
240–249	2	0	2
250–259	1	0	1
Total	170	41	211

Table 6.3 gives the weight of the victims. Males weighed in excess of 170 lb in 110(52.1%) cases, while 30(14.2%) of the women weighed less than 130 lb.

LEVEL OF INJURY

Table 6.4 reports the level of injury to the spinal column as reported in the medical records. Of the total injuries, 124(58.8%) involved the C-5 and C-5, 6 levels and where indicated in the medical record were of the flexion type.

SOURCE OF INITIAL SWIMMING AND DIVING INSTRUCTION

Table 6.5 indicates the age the victim learned to swim. It is very interesting to note that 192(91.0%) had learned to swim before the age of 8 years.

Table 6.6 indicates where the victim had received his initial diving instruction. Only 44 (20.9%) received any formal diving instruction. Slightly more than half (54.5%) were self-taught, and approximately one quarter (52, 24.6%) indicated that they had received instruction from their parents or another family member.

TABLE 6.4
Level of Injury

Level	Males	Females	Total
C–1	1	1	2
C–1, 2	2	0	2
C–3, 4	2	0	2
C–4	6	0	6
C–4, 5	19	3	22
C–5	50	13	63
C–5, 6	47	14	61
C–4, 5, 6	1	0	1
C–6	14	1	15
C–6, 7	16	5	21
C–7	2	0	2
C–7, T–1	2	0	2
T–1	1	0	1
T–1, 2, 3	1	0	1
Some neurological impairment	4	2	6
Fractured skull	1	1	2
Brain hemorrhage	1	1	2
Total	170	41	211

TABLE 6.5
Age Victim Learned to Swim

Age	Number
1–4	60
5–8	132
9–12	16
13 and over	3
Total	211

TABLE 6.6
Source of Initial Diving Instruction

Source	Number
Self-taught	115
Parent or family member	52
City recreation department	24
American Red Cross	12
YMCA	6
School or college	2
Total	211

TABLE 6.7
Pool Ownership

Owner	Number
Residential	71
Apartment/condominium	55
Motel/Hotel	54
Municipality(city, county)	12
Commercial	7
Voluntary agency	6
Private/country club	4
Others	2
Total	211

POOL FACILITIES

POOL OWNERSHIP

Table 6.7 identifies the owner of the property or facility where the accident occurred. Of the 211 pools involved, 71(33.6%) were owned by individual families. These are commonly classified as residential pools.

What was surprising was the number that were owned and operated by motels/hotels and by apartments/condominiums. Combined, these two categories accounted for 109(51.7%) of the pools. When the number of residential pools are added, the total of 180 pools represents 85.3% of the accident sites.

LOCATION BY STATE

Table 6.8 reveals that 208(98.6%) accidents occurred in 41 different states; and one each, in the Virgin Islands, Canada, and Mexico.

POOL SHAPES

Table 6.9 identifies the various pool shapes. Conventional rectangular pools represented 71(33.6%). A total of 56(26.5%) were of the hopper-bottom design where the deep portion (diving area) had a truncated end and sides, in essence producing a pool comparable to an inverted pyramid. These pools all had a vinyl liner as the water container. Of particular interest is the fact that there were 12(5.7%) distinctly different, identifiable designs of pools plus the 14(6.6%) free-form shapes, which invariably incorporated elements from many of the traditional pool designs.

BASIN FINISH

Table 6.10 indicates the basin composition of the accident pool. The majority (149, 70.6%) were either gunite or poured concrete.

POOL MARKINGS

Table 6.11 indicates the frequency and type of pool markings that were present at the time of the accident. A surprising 76(36.0%) pools had no depth markers at any location on or around the pool. Even fewer (44, 20.9%) of the pools had any type of bottom markings. The least common indicator of depth was the presence of a lifeline in only 28(13.3%) of the pool.

TABLE 6.8
Location by State

State	Number	State	Number
Florida	20	Kentucky	3
California	16	Oklahoma	3
Illinois	14	Connecticut	3
Texas	14	Kansas	2
Pennsylvania	11	Mississippi	2
Michigan	10	Nevada	2
Iowa	9	New Jersey	2
Ohio	9	Rhode Island	2
Arizona	7	Wisconsin	2
Indiana	7	Wyoming	2
Louisiana	7	Alaska	1
Massachusetts	6	Idaho	1
Minnesota	6	Maine	1
Virginia	6	Montana	1
Alabama	5	Nebraska	1
Missouri	5	New Mexico	1
Colorado	4	North Carolina	1
Georgia	4	Vermont	1
Hawaii	4	Washington	1
Maryland	4	Virgin Islands	1
New York	4	Quebec	1
Tennessee	4	Mexico	1
		Total	211

TABLE 6.9
Pool Shapes

Shape	Number
Conventional, rectangular	71
Hopper bottom	56
"L" or Lazy "L"	30
Kidney	18
Free form	14
Round/circular	8
"T"	5
Fan	3
Clover leaf	2
Pear	1
Double kidney	1
Half moon	1
Square	1
Total	211

DEPTH OF WATER AT IMPACT

Table 6.12 contains the estimated depth of water where the victim contacted the bottom of the pool. The depth between 3 ft 1 in. and 3 ft 6 in. produced the most injuries (67, 31.8%). The five (2.4%)

TABLE 6.10
Basin Composition

Finish	NUMBER
Gunite	84
Poured concrete	65
Vinyl liner	59
Concrete wall/sand bottom	1
Aluminum	1
Fiberglass	1
Total	211

TABLE 6.11
Pool Markings

Marking	Yes	No	Total
Depth markings	135	76	211
Bottom markings	44	167	211
Lifeline in place	28	183	211

TABLE 6.12
Depth of Water at Impact

Depth (ft/in.)	Number
0/0	5
0/5–0/6	0
0/7–1/0	0
1/1–1/6	0
1/7–2/0	1
2/1–2/6	8
2/7–3/0	65
3/1–3/6	67
3/7–4/0	39
4/1–4/6	17
4/7–5/0	6
5/1–5/6	1
5/7–6/0	1
6/1–6/6	1
Total	211

recorded at the zero depth were those who struck the pool deck or were struck by another diver. Eight (4.0%) occurred in water depths ranging from 2 ft 1 in. to 2 ft 6 in. The most significant statistic is that 185 (87.7%) of the injuries resulted from the diver striking the bottom in water that was 4 ft or less in depth. As shown in Table 6.12, only three (1.4%) victims struck the bottom of the pool where the depth of water was more than 5 ft 1 in. All the dives occurred in hopper-bottom pools with the victims diving across the deep end of the pool and striking the sloping wall that went down from the 3-ft-vertical wall at an angle of 45 degrees to the bottom of the pool. This sloping wall is what the victims struck (see Figure 6.1).

It is important to understand that the method employed to arrive at the estimated depth came from two sources: first, where the victim was spotted by other swimmers present after striking the bottom; and second, when there were eyewitnesses to the dive. Where the impact point occurred on the slope of the bottom, a range was established for both the entry point and the angle of underwater trajectory; then a mean calculated. This was the figure that was recorded.

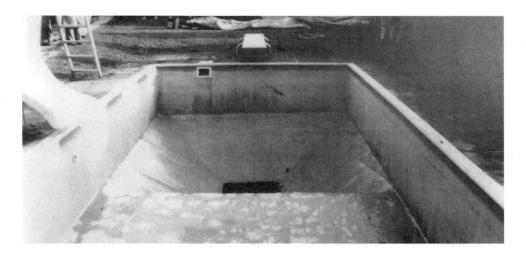

FIGURE 6.1 Hopper-bottom pool showing the sloping sides in the deep end of the pool, which makes a dive across the pool dangerous.

TABLE 6.13
Clarity of Water

Clarity	Number
Empty	1
Clear	164
Semiturbid	41
Turbid	5
Total	211

TABLE 6.14
Lighting and Weather

Factor	Yes	No	Total
Lighting	87	124	211
Weather	3	208	211

ENVIRONMENTAL FACTORS

CLARITY OF WATER

Table 6.13 represents the clarity of the water at the time of the accident. It was the judgment of witnesses that the water in 164(77.7%) of the cases was clear, semiturbid in 41(19.4%), and turbid (cloudy) in only 5(2.4%) instances. In one case the pool was empty.

LIGHTING AND WEATHER

The prevailing conditions at the time of the accident are presented in Table 6.14. While weather was a factor in only 3(1.4%) of the accidents, pool lighting (i.e., illumination in and around the pool) was found to be a factor in 87(41.2%) of the cases, which indicates the dives were made at nighttime.

PRE- AND POSTACCIDENT EVENTS

VICTIM: GUEST OR OWNER

Of the 211 accidents, only 5(2.4%) of the victims were members of the household, or owners or staff members of the motels/hotels or apartments/condominiums. The balance 206(97.6%), as shown in Table 6.15, were guests or visitors to the pool.

TIME AND DAY OF THE ACCIDENT

Table 6.16 highlights that the afternoon hours between 2 and 6 P.M. represented 93(44.1%) of the accidents. Evening hours between 6 P.M. and midnight accounted for 80(37.9%) cases. Three days—Friday, Saturday, and Sunday—accounted for 128(60.7%) accidents.

YEAR AND MONTH OF ACCIDENT

Table 6.17 lists the months in which the accidents occurred. As anticipated, more accidents occurred in the summer months of June, July and August, representing 125(59.2%) of the total. Table 6.18 records the years in which the accidents occurred.

VICTIM'S VISITS TO THE POOL

Tables 6.19 through 6.21 contain the tabulation of the frequency of the victim's visits and the number of dives made at the pool where his injury occurred.

Table 6.19 indicates that in 141 (66.8%) of the cases the victim was visiting the pool for the first time. This is the most significant fact when considering who is at greatest risk.

TABLE 6.15
Victim: Guest or Owner

Victim	Number
Guest	206
Owner	5
Total	211

TABLE 6.16
Time and Day of Accident

Time Interval	Mon.	Tue.	Wed.	Thu.	Fri.	Sat.	Sun.	Total
12:00–01:59 A.M.	3	0	0	0	3	4	4	14
02:00–03:59 A.M.	1	1	2	1	1	1	1	8
04:00–05:59 A.M.	1	0	0	0	0	0	0	1
06:00–07:59 A.M.	0	0	0	0	0	1	0	1
08:00–09:59 A.M.	0	0	0	0	0	0	0	0
10:00–11:59 A.M.	0	0	0	1	1	1	1	4
12:00–01:59 P.M.	1	1	1	1	1	3	2	10
02:00–03:59 P.M.	1	3	1	3	2	13	15	38
04:00–05:59 P.M.	7	10	2	6	12	8	10	55
06:00–07:59 P.M.	2	2	1	1	4	4	4	18
08:00–09:59 P.M.	2	2	2	3	6	6	8	29
10:00–11:59 P.M.	3	1	13	4	4	4	4	33
TOTAL	21	20	22	20	34	45	49	211

TABLE 6.17
Month of Accident

Month	Number	Month	Number
January	3	July	53
February	10	August	36
March	9	September	12
April	16	October	6
May	20	November	6
June	36	December	4
		Total	211

TABLE 6.18
Year of Accident

Year	Number	Year	Number
Before 1970	1	1981	18
1970	5	1982	23
1971	4	1983	26
1972	9	1984	14
1973	3	1985	11
1974	5	1986	7
1975	8	1987	8
1976	13	1988	8
1977	9	1989	5
1978	7	1990	0
1979	9	1991	1
1980	17	Total	211

TABLE 6.19
Victim's Visits to the Pool

Visits	First	Prior	Total
None	141	0	141
One or two	0	23	23
Three or more	0	47	47
Total	141	70	211

TABLE 6.20
Dives Made on Prior Visits

Dives	Number
One dive	14
Two to three Dives	7
Four or more	49
Total	70

Dives Made on Prior Visits

Only 70(33.2%) of the victims had visited the pool previously, with 56(26.5%) of those having made more than one previous dive (see Table 6.20).

Dives Made on Day of Accident

Table 6.21 reveals 139(65.9%) were injured on the first dive the victim made into the pool.

TABLE 6.21
Dives Made on Day of Accident

Dives	Number
First	139
Two to Three	48
Four or more	24
Total	211

TABLE 6.22
Position of Arms/Hands at Entry

Position	Number
In front	191
No recollection	8
At side (sailor's dive)	5
Not applicable	6
Around knees	1
Total	211

TABLE 6.23
Location of Dive

Location	Number
Dived from shallow end of pool	62
Side of pool in shallow end	48
Side of shallow end toward deep end	40
Deep side toward shallow end	9
Deep end toward shallow end	9
Deep side across pool	4
Roof of house	4
Sundeck 3' high	2
3rd floor balcony	1
Slide into shallow end	16
Slide into deep end	1
Slider hit side of slide	2
Fell off top of slide	1
Thrown in pool from deck of pool	3
Did reverse cannonball	2
Struck underwater steps while swimming underwater	2
Fell and hit head on coping	2
Did back dive	1
Hit outcropping on stone deck	1
Struck by another swimmer	1
Total	211

POSITION OF ARMS/HANDS AT ENTRY

As Table 6.22 reveals, 191(90.5%) of the divers reportedly had their arms and hands in front of them as they made their dives. Five (2.4%) victims had their arms at their sides, as in a "sailor's dive." Six (2.8%) were injured where the hands played no role in the accident, while eight (3.8%) could not remember where their arms were and no one saw the dive.

LOCATION OF DIVE

There were 20 different locations where the dives took place as indicated in Table 6.23.

The shallow portion of the pool accounted for most of the accidents, which included 16(7.6%) victims injured while going down water slides located at the shallow end of the pool and 3(1.4%) victims that were thrown into the pool by other swimmers.

TABLE 6.24
Type of Social Setting

Setting	Number
Informal	171
Formal	40
Total	211

TABLE 6.25
Substance Abuse

Substance	Yes	No	Total
Alcohol	99	112	211
Drugs	4	207	211

There were several unusual accident types. Among these were a dive into a pool that was empty; sliders who fell off the top of the slide and struck the coping of the pool; a dive from a balcony three floors above the pool; a swimmer who, while in the water, was struck by a diver coming off a 3-m-high springboard; and three divers who made their dive from the roof of a garage.

TYPE OF SOCIAL SETTING

The type of social gathering involved is indicated in Table 6.24. Only 40 (19.0%) were attending a formal party where invitations had been sent. Most of these were company parties. The other 171 (81.0%) were participating in a type of informal social activity, most of which were impromptu get-togethers of people ranging in number from 3 to 30.

SUBSTANCE ABUSE

Table 6.25 indicates that of the 211 victims, 99 (46.9%) had consumed some form of alcoholic beverage (mostly beer). Blood alcohol tests were taken in only a few of the cases. The residential pool usually involving a party was the predominant scene where alcohol was consumed. Only four (1.9%) victims admitted or were identified by others to have consumed any form of drugs on the day of their accident. However, in ten (4.7%) other cases there was evidence that drugs were on the premises where the pool was located.

SAFETY AND SUPERVISION

POSTED RULES AND WARNING SIGNS

Warning signs prohibiting diving were present in only 18 (8.5%) of the pools where the accident occurred, as shown in Table 6.26. In 193 (91.5%) of the cases, the victims did not have the benefit of warnings against diving at the location where they made their fateful dives.

LIFEGUARD ON DUTY

Lifeguards were on duty in only 52 (24.6%) of the pools involved in these accidents, as shown in Table 6.27. These pools were invariably at public (city or county), school, or club facilities.

RESCUE PROCEDURES

PERSON MAKING RESCUE

Table 6.28 identifies the person who made the initial rescue of the victim from the pool. Most 156 (73.9%) were rescued by friends or other swimmers who were nearby. Lifeguards performed only 35 (16.6%) rescues.

TABLE 6.26			
Posted Rules and Warning Signs			
Instructions	**Yes**	**No**	**Total**
Posted rules	137	74	211
Warning signs	18	193	211

TABLE 6.27	
Lifeguard on Duty	
Lifeguard	**Number**
Yes	52
No	159
Total	211

TABLE 6.28	
Person Making Rescue	
Rescuer	**Number**
Friends	156
Lifeguard	35
Self	9
Emergency medical services (EMS)	8
Security guard	3
Total	211

TABLE 6.29			
Use of Spineboard and CPR			
Technique	**Yes**	**No**	**Total**
Spineboard used	16	195	211
CPR administered	22	189	211

USE OF SPINEBOARD AND CARDIOPULMONARY RESUSCITATION

A very disturbing fact, as revealed in Table 6.29, indicates that rescuers used a spineboard in only 16(7.6%) cases. This means that the vast majority of victims were lifted, pulled, or dragged out of the water by friends who, in general, were not aware of the injury. Cardiopulmonary resuscitation (CPR) was administered to only 22(10.4%) of the victims because most never lost consciousness.

This further implies that the rescue of the victim was probably within a minute or two from the time he was injured. Paramedics were used in all but nine (4.3%) of the cases to transport the victim to the nearest hospital.

CONCLUSIONS

As the term implies, the inground pools are those where the ground was excavated for installation. We separated the injuries occurring from aboveground pools (Chapter 5), springboards (Chapter 7), and starting blocks (Chapter 8). Ownership of these pools ranges from homeowners to agencies, as shown in Table 6.7. These pools can be of a variety of sizes and shapes as shown in Table 6.9. The conclusions the Editorial Board arrived at as to the causes of the 211 dives made into inground pools are as follows:

1. The most disturbing fact is that in all (208, 98.6%) but 3(1.4%) of the 211 injuries, the depth of water where the victims struck the bottom was under 5 ft; and in most (185, 87.7%), the depth of water was 4 ft or less. See Figure 6.2 that shows six divers' heads coming in contact with the simulated bottom.
2. Of the 211 pools in the study, 109(51.7%) were owned either by apartment/condominiums (55, 26.1%), or by motels/hotels(54, 25.6%). These pools were operated without lifeguards, and only six of the pools had any signs prohibiting diving in the shallow portion of the pool.
3. The hopper-bottom pools and the spoon-shaped pools are, in our opinion, exceedingly dangerous because there are no markings (lines) on the bottom to indicate to the diver the depth of water or the contour of the pool bottom. Most of these are residential-type pools.

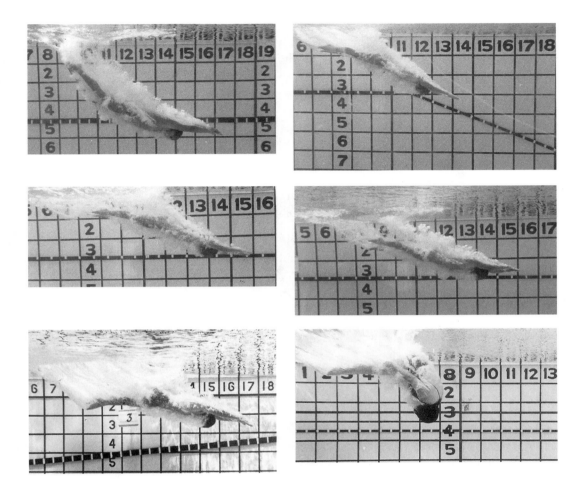

FIGURE 6.2 Underwater photos of six divers who dove off a 6-ft-high deck. The arms and head are incorrectly located with hands providing no protection for the head.

4. It was shocking to find that 41(66.8%) of the 211 injuries happened on the victim's first dive into the pool.
5. Alcohol was a factor in 99(46.9%) of the injuries, but none of the victims were below the legal age limit.
6. There were 20 different locations in the pool where the injuries occurred, but one fact stood out. All were in the shallow portion of the pool (under 5 ft).
7. We interviewed more than 100 of the victims and they all said, "I didn't believe I would get hurt. If someone had told me not to dive, I would not have done so."
8. Another disturbing fact was that most of the injured were rescued and pulled or dragged out of the pool by friends with no spineboards being used.
9. We are convinced that pools have to be designed more safely and managed more effectively. This implies that whenever home pool owners invite people over for a swim in their pools they take on the responsibility not only to supervise them but also to warn them about what they must not do. Most of the victims were either a guest of a homeowner or a guest at a motel/hotel.

Figure 6.3 illustrates the position of the diver above water making a safe shallow dive, and Figure 6.4 shows the body angle underwater that is safe. Figure 6.5 illustrates the extremely dangerous angle of the diver's body as he enters the pool. This position requires immediate raising of the head and arching of the back to avoid head contact with the bottom.

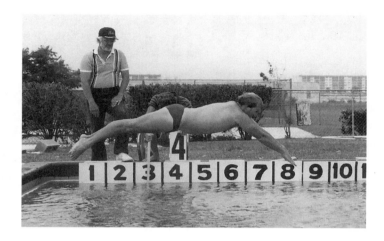

FIGURE 6.3 Illustrates the safe body alignment of diver while above water from a deck dive.

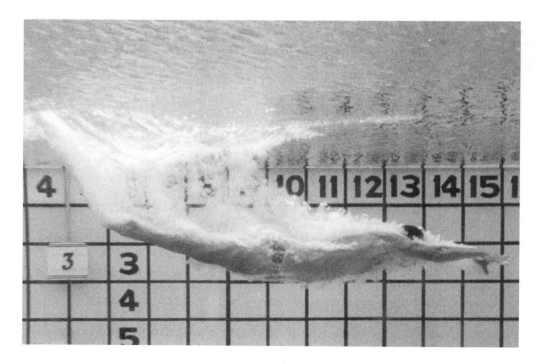

FIGURE 6.4 Shows safe body alignment of diver underwater in a dive from the pool deck.

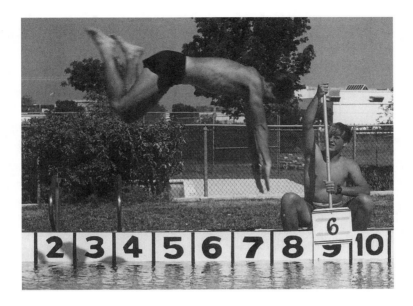

FIGURE 6.5 A dangerous dive from the deck following a run to the edge of the pool with the diver achieving too much height. This increases the entry velocity.

7 Springboard/Jumpboard Diving Accidents

INTRODUCTION

This chapter contains the data for 92 cases that occurred from people diving off springboards or jumpboards into inground swimming pools. As the name implies, springboards are those that derive their spring from the board's flexibility, while the jumpboards utilize coil springs or cantilever devices to obtain the spring to project the diver up and out. Whenever springboard diving is mentioned, it includes jumpboards as well. Excluded from this chapter are 211 dives made into inground pools from decks and adjacent structures that are covered in Chapter 6, and dives from starting blocks that are presented in Chapter 8.

The 92 cases represent 20.9% of the 440 pool cases. The data, once collected, were then computerized and tables were developed and placed under the following categories:

- Victims
- Pool Facilities and boards
- Environmental factors
- Pre- and postaccident events
- Safety and supervision
- Rescue procedures

BACKGROUND

There are three basic areas that may affect the performance of people diving from springboards— human, environmental, and mechanical. (A detailed description of the mechanics of diving is presented in Chapter 10.)

HUMAN FACTORS

- Physical attributes of the diver: height, weight, and strength of arms and legs
- Physiological factors such as visual acuity, fatigue, illness, and drug and alcohol consumption
- Ability and agility of the diver including athletic ability, experience in diving, and training under qualified leadership
- Psychological factors such as social setting, peer pressure, and fear

ENVIRONMENTAL FACTORS

- Configuration of the bottom of the pool
- Coefficient of friction of the pool bottom surface

- Depth of water in the diver's landing area
- Bottom markings
- Composition and flexibility of the board (wood, laminated wood, metal, aluminum, or fiberglass)
- Length and width of the board
- Position and type of fulcrum
- Type of stand or mounting for board
- Artificial illumination of pool and area
- Position of the sun
- Glare on water surface
- Wind (particularly lateral winds)

MECHANICS OF DIVING

- Speed of the approach
- Horizontal distance of the hurdle
- Height of the hurdle
- Board depression
- Leg flexion
- Angle of the takeoff
- Lift of the arms
- Angle of entry into the water
- Alignment of the body underwater
- Position of the head, hands, and arms underwater
- Underwater trajectory of the diver
- Changes in the body alignment underwater

EVOLUTION OF DIVING BOARDS

Competitive Diving Boards

Springboards employed in competitive diving have evolved from the one-piece Douglas fir board that emerged in the 1920s to the advanced technology aluminum boards of today. There is no comparison between the wooden boards of the 1930s and today's aluminum boards. These high-performance boards are used at all major championships throughout the world. Although the competitive rules for diving do not specify that the board must be constructed of any particular material, it is widely accepted that the highest performance board is made of extruded aluminum. Therefore, competitive divers and their coaches settled mainly on one type of springboard—the aluminum board measuring 16 ft in length and 20 in. wide, although some manufacturers produced 14 ft boards. Figure 7.1 demonstrates the great flexibility of the 16-ft-long aluminum competitive springboard.

Another area of agreement among officials is that the fulcrum on which the board sets must be of the adjustable type. Figure 7.2 illustrates a 3-m-high board with an adjustable fulcrum mounted on a concrete platform.

Competitive diving appears to have settled on a 16-ft-long board with very little variation between the kinds of stands that are acceptable. Boards for primarily recreational use have no set model. They range in length from 3 to 14 ft with at least 36 different types of mounting.

Recreational Diving Boards

It was obvious that these 14- and 16-ft-high-performance springboards were not safe to place on residential or smaller type pools designed primarily to accommodate recreational swimmers. At the beginning there was nothing to guide board manufacturers with respect to the kind of boards

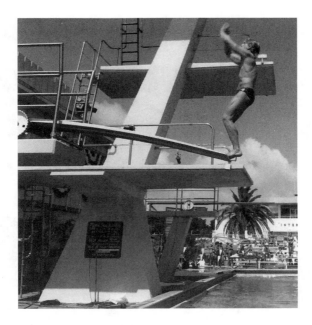

FIGURE 7.1 Demonstration of the flexibility of a 16-ft-long aluminum springboard used in diving competition.

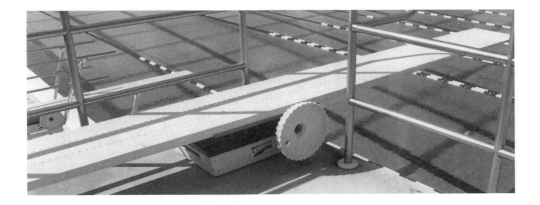

FIGURE 7.2 Adjustable fulcrum used in competitive diving.

suitable for smaller pools, except their imaginations. Unfortunately, for some reason they felt compelled to offer the customer a variety of boards and stands ranging from 3 to 14 ft long. Few tried to compete with the manufacturers of aluminum boards. Most noncompetitive boards today are made with a wood core that is covered with fiberglass.

Then came the revolution. People wanted spring in their boards. The wooden boards with a fixed fulcrum, as shown in Figure 7.3, did not have much spring. Manufacturers tried moving the fulcrum back, which increased the spring, but because of the added bend to the board when used by divers, the wood core would crack and sometimes break prematurely. Correcting this problem was a challenge to board manufacturers. They concluded that they had to get the spring by some means other than the bending (flexibility) of a wood core. Thus "jumpboards" were born. These boards utilize coil springs as shown in Figure 7.4 and other designs as shown in Figure 7.5(a). Figure 7.5(b) illustrates that the spring no longer is derived from the board, but instead from the two 6-in.

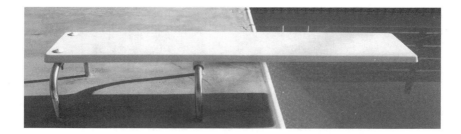

FIGURE 7.3 Wooden springboard with fixed fulcrum.

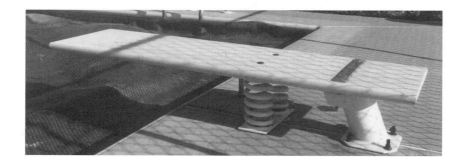

FIGURE 7.4 Jump board using coil springs to provide the diver with greater spring.

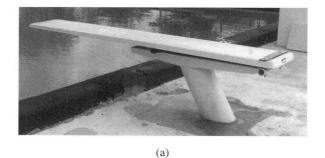

(a)

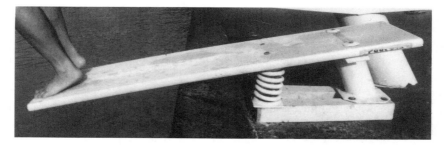

(b)

FIGURE 7.5 Two other diving board stands that illustrate other methods used to obtain spring. Note that the springboard in (b) does not bend. Spring is derived from the coil.

coils located under the board. The heavier the diver is, the greater the spring. The coil spring is quite a bit faster in its recovery after being depressed than conventional boards. Figure 7.6 shows the height that a diver may reach from an 8-ft-long board. Figure 7.7 illustrates a type of board mount where the spring is generated by steel straps.

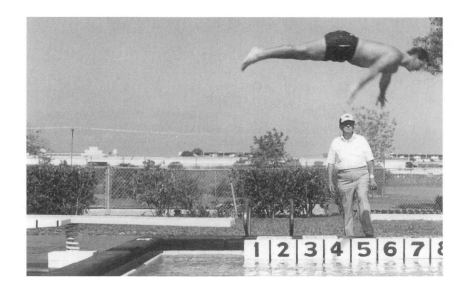

FIGURE 7.6 Illustrates height diver can achieve from an 8-ft-long board with coil spring.

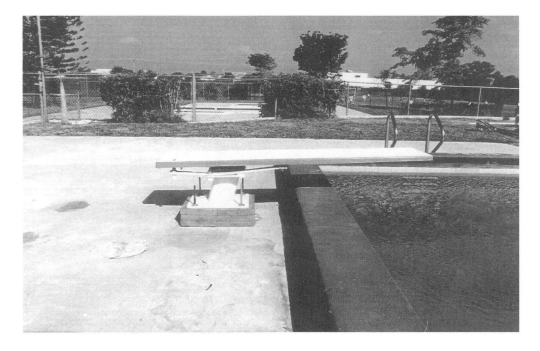

FIGURE 7.7 Illustrates the type of board mount where the spring is generated by steel straps.

VICTIMS

AGE AND SEX

Table 7.1 gives the age and sex of the victims. Only 6(6.5%) of the 92 victims were female. The table also reveals that 39(42.4%) of the victims ranged in age from 22 to 42, which is contrary to public opinion that the majority of injuries involve teenagers. An additional finding that is contrary to the stereotypical victim is that 20(21.7%) of the victims were or had been married, and many had children.

TABLE 7.1
Age and Sex of Victims

Ages	Males	Females	Total
10–12	0	2	2
13–15	7	3	10
16–18	26	0	26
19–21	15	0	15
22–24	14	0	14
25–27	5	0	5
28–30	6	1	7
31–33	7	0	7
34–36	3	0	3
37–39	1	0	1
40–42	2	0	2
Total	86	6	92

TABLE 7.2
Height of Victims

Height (ft/in.)	Males	Females	Total
5/0	1	1	2
5/1	0	0	0
5/2	0	1	1
5/3	0	0	0
5/4	0	2	2
5/5	1	2	3
5/6	2	0	2
5/7	6	0	6
5/8	8	0	8
5/9	6	0	6
5/10	10	0	10
5/11	11	0	11
6/0	20	0	20
6/1	9	0	9
6/2	5	0	5
6/3	2	0	2
6/4	3	0	3
6/5	2	0	2
Total	86	6	92

TABLE 7.3
Weight of Victims

Weight (lb)	Males	Females	Total
90–99	1	0	1
100–109	1	1	2
110–119	1	3	4
120–129	1	0	1
130–139	3	2	5
140–149	9	0	9
150–159	4	0	4
160–169	10	0	10
170–179	24	0	24
180–189	12	0	12
190–199	5	0	5
200–209	7	0	7
210–219	2	0	2
220–229	3	0	3
230–239	2	0	2
240–249	1	0	1
Total	86	6	92

HEIGHT AND WEIGHT

Tables 7.2 and 7.3 give the height and weight of the victims. With respect to height, 62(67.4%) were 5 ft 10 in. or more. It is significant that 56(60.9%) of the victims weighed in excess of 170 lb. Males are, without a doubt, at the greatest risk in diving accidents.

LEVEL OF INJURY

Table 7.4 indicates the level and type of injury sustained by the victims based on a review of the medical records in each case. All (85, 92.4%) but 7(7.6%) of the 92 victims had complete or incomplete quadriplegia; 6(6.5%) were diagnosed with some neurological impairment. The most frequent injury, representing 54(58.7%) of the victims, was a fracture of the spine at the C-5 or C-5, 6 level.

SOURCE OF INITIAL SWIMMING AND DIVING INSTRUCTION

Tables 7.5 and 7.6 identify the early swimming and diving background of the victims, which indicate when they first learned to swim and the source of their instructions in diving. Table 7.5 indicates that 85(92.4%) of the individuals learned to swim by the time they were 8 years old.

TABLE 7.4
Level of Injury

Level	Males	Females	Total
C–2, 3	1	0	1
C–3, 4	2	0	2
C–4	2	0	2
C–4, 5	10	0	10
C–5	28	1	29
C–5, 6	24	1	25
C–6	5	0	5
C–6, 7	7	1	8
C–7	1	0	1
T–1, 2	1	0	1
T–6, 7	1	0	1
Some neurological impairment	4	2	6
Fractured jaw	0	1	1
Total	86	6	92

TABLE 7.5
Age Victim Learned to Swim

Age	Number
1–4	25
5–8	60
9–12	6
13 and over	1
Total	92

TABLE 7.6
Source of Initial Diving Instruction

Source	Number
Self-taught	52
Parent or family member	24
American Red Cross	6
School or college	4
YMCA	4
City recreation department	2
Total	92

POOL FACILITIES AND BOARDS

POOL OWNERSHIP

Residential pools were the site of 52(56.5%) of the accidents, as shown in Table 7.7. When the number of pools located at motels/hotels and apartments/condominiums are added to the residential total, the percentage of accidents associated with living facilities reaches 80(87.0%).

LOCATION BY STATE

Table 7.8 reveals that 90(97.8%) of the accidents occurred in 29 different states; 1 each occurred in Washington, D.C., and in the Virgin Islands. Florida had the highest number of accidents (11, 12.0%) followed closely by Illinois and Pennsylvania.

POOL SHAPES

Table 7.9 identifies the shape of the pools involved in the accidents. Rectangular pools numbered 62(67.4%); 10(10.9%) were kidney shaped; 6(6.5%) were "L" shaped; and 8(8.7%) others were a modified "L."

TABLE 7.7
Pool Ownership

Owner	Number
Residential	52
Motel/hotel	18
Apartment/condominium	10
Municipality (city, county)	8
High school/college	2
Voluntary agency	1
Private/country club	1
Total	92

TABLE 7.8
Location by State

State	Number	State	Number
Florida	11	South Carolina	2
Pennsylvania	10	Wisconsin	2
Illinois	10	Alabama	1
New Jersey	6	Colorado	1
Texas	6	Connecticut	1
Arizona	4	Kentucky	1
California	4	Massachusetts	1
Indiana	4	Missouri	1
New York	4	New Hampshire	1
Michigan	3	Tennessee	1
Kansas	3	Virginia	1
Louisiana	2	Washington	1
Minnesota	2	West Virginia	1
Nevada	2	Washington, D.C.	1
Ohio	2	Virgin Islands	1
Rhode Island	2	Total	92

TABLE 7.9
Pool Shapes

Shape	Number
Conventional, rectangular	62
Kidney	10
Modified "L"	8
"L"	6
"T"	3
Circular/round	2
Free form	1
Total	92

TABLE 7.10
Basin Composition

Finish	Number
Vinyl liner	43
Gunite	33
Poured concrete	16
Total	92

TABLE 7.11
Board Type by Owner

Pool owner	3m	2m	1m	<1m	Total
Residential	0	0	0	57	57
Motel/hotel	5	1	2	7	15
City/county	8	0	0	0	8
Aptartment/Condominium	0	0	4	4	8
High school	2	0	0	0	2
Agency	0	0	1	0	1
Country club	0	0	1	0	1
Total	15	1	8	68	92

BASIN FINISH

Table 7.10 lists the types of basin finish. Slightly more than half (49, 53.3%) were concrete or gunite while slightly less than half (43, 46.7%) had vinyl liners.

BOARD TYPE

Tables 7.11 and 7.12 contain data that are unique to springboards and jumpboards. As Table 7.11 indicates, 15(16.3%) of the injuries resulted from dives off of 3-m-high (10-ft) springboards. Of these, five (5.4%) were located at motel/hotel pools; eight (8.7%), at city or county pools; and two (2.2%), at school pools. Of interest is the fact that all the 3-m-boards were removed after the injury. All the boards located at residential pools were low boards with a height above the water between 18 and 26 in. Table 7.12 gives a breakdown of all 92 pools with respect to the board length, and the height of the board above the water surface.

BOTTOM PROFILE OF POOL

Table 7.13 indicates the pool bottom profile. A spoon-shaped bottom profile was found in 48(52.2%) of the cases while 44(47.8%) were hopper-bottom types.

SITE OF DIVE

Table 7.14 indicates the type of diving equipment from which the dive was made and the nature of the dive involved in the accident. Dives from low, noncompetitive size boards represented 72(78.3%) of the accidents.

POOL MARKINGS

Table 7.15 shows that depth markers in the diving portion of the pool were present in 36(39.1%) of the cases. These were mostly residential pools. Only 7(7.6%) of the 92 pools studied had any bottom markings in the diving area of the pool. These were all competitive-type pools. Only 22(23.9%) of the pools had a lifeline in place at the time of the accident. One purpose of the lifeline is to indicate to the diver where the breakpoint (start of the slope down to the deep portion of the pool) was located.

DEPTH OF WATER

Table 7.16 indicates the maximum depth of water. In 77(83.7%) of the pools, the maximum water depth was less than 9 ft. Table 7.17 contains the estimated depth of water where the victim contacted the bottom.

TABLE 7.12
Type of Board and Height from Water

Board	Length (ft)	Height	Number
Jumpboards	3–8	13–22 in.	17
Springboards			
Pedestal	8–10	22–27 in.	23
Pipe "U" frame	8–12	24–26 in.	29
1-m Stand	14	30 in.	1
	16	36–39 in.	8
2-m Stand	14	2 m	1
3-m Stand	16	3 m	12
	14	3 m	1
Total			92

TABLE 7.13
Bottom Profile of Deep End

Profile	Number
Spoon	48
Hopper	44
Total	92

TABLE 7.14
Site of Dive

Dive Description	Number	Total
Low Boards 18–30 in. Above Water		72
Running dives		
Plain front from springboard with bounce on end	51	
Plain front from jumpboard	8	
$1\frac{1}{2}$ somersault from springboard	4	
Standing dives		
Plain front from springboard	5	
Plain front from jumpboard	2	
Back dive from springboard	2	
3-m-High Springboards		15
Plain running front dive	10	
$1\frac{1}{2}$ somersault	2	
Person in water struck by diver	3	
Other Types		5
Dives through inner tube from low board (26 in.)	3	
Fell from 1-meter dive stand and struck concrete deck	1	
Struck sidewall of pool	1	
Total		92

TABLE 7.15
Pool Markings

Marking	Yes	No	Total
Depth markings	36	56	92
Bottom markings	7	85	92
Lifeline in place	22	70	92

TABLE 7.16
Maximum Depth of Water

Depth (ft/in.)	Number
Below 6/0	2
6/1–7/0	7
7/1–8/0	36
8/1–9/0	32
9/1–10/0	11
10/1–11/0	2
Above 11/0	2
Total	92

TABLE 7.17
Depth of Water at Impact

Depth (ft/in.)	Number
3/0 and under	6
3/1–3/6	1
3/7–4/0	8
4/1–4/6	18
4/7–5/0	32
5/1–5/6	13
5/7–6/0	8
6/1–6/7	4
6/7–7/0	2
Total	92

TABLE 7.18 Clarity of Water	
Clarity	**Number**
Empty	0
Clear	80
Semiturbid	0
Turbid	12
Total	92

TABLE 7.19 Lighting and Weather			
Factor	**Yes**	**No**	**Total**
Lighting	20	72	92
Weather	0	92	92

The data employed to arrive at the estimated depth came from two sources: first, where the victim was spotted by other swimmers present after striking the bottom, and second, when there were eyewitnesses to the dive. Where the impact point occurred on the slope of the bottom, a range was established for both the entry point and the angle of underwater trajectory, and a mean was calculated. This was the figure that was recorded. Those accidents recorded at 3 ft or below involved those victims who struck the pool deck or were struck by another diver.

A very disturbing fact was that all the victims struck the bottom of the pool at a water depth that was less than 7 ft deep and most struck the upslope of the bottom of the pool at a perpendicular angle.

ENVIRONMENTAL FACTORS

CLARITY OF WATER

In 80(87.0%) of the accidents, witnesses indicated that they thought the water was clear. The criterion used was whether the bottom drain of the pool was visible (Table 7.18).

LIGHTING AND WEATHER

Table 7.19 presents two environmental factors, namely, pool lighting and weather factors. In only 20(21.7%) of the diving accidents was lighting considered to be a factor. However, no light meter readings were taken. The judgment of witnesses present at the time of the accident, the victim, and the investigator were the basis for determining whether lighting was a factor. The data showed that weather conditions at the time of the incident were not a factor and did not contribute to the accident in any way.

PRE- AND POSTACCIDENT EVENTS

Information was collected about the activities related to the pre- and postaccident events, as well as the circumstances directly related to the accident.

VICTIM: GUEST OR OWNER

Of those injured, 86(93.5%) were guests of homeowners or visitors to pools located at motel/hotel, apartment/condominium, or public facilities. Of the 92 injured in residential pools, 6(6.5%) were members of the households. None of the victims was a trespasser (Table 7.20).

TIME AND DAY OF ACCIDENT

Table 7.21 shows the time and day when accidents occurred. Friday, Saturday, and Sunday accounted for 53(57.6%) of the accidents. The daylight hours between 2 and 6 P.M. accounted for 51(55.4%)

TABLE 7.20
Victim: Guest or Owner

Victim	Number
Guest	86
Owner	6
Total	92

TABLE 7.21
Time and Day of Accident

Time Interval	Mon.	Tue.	Wed.	Thu.	Fri.	Sat.	Sun.	Total
12:00–01:59 A.M.	0	0	0	0	0	1	1	2
02:00–03:59 A.M.	0	0	0	0	0	1	2	3
04:00–05:59 A.M.	0	0	0	0	0	0	0	0
06:00–07:59 A.M.	1	0	0	0	0	0	0	1
08:00–09:59 A.M.	0	0	0	0	0	0	0	0
10:00–11:59 A.M.	0	0	0	0	0	0	0	0
12:00–01:59 P.M.	0	1	1	2	1	1	1	7
02:00–03:59 P.M.	1	1	2	6	3	3	3	19
04:00–05:59 P.M.	1	0	8	5	6	6	6	32
06:00–07:59 P.M.	0	1	1	1	1	4	4	12
08:00–09:59 P.M.	1	1	1	1	1	2	1	8
10:00–11:59 P.M.	1	0	1	1	1	2	2	8
Total	5	4	14	16	13	20	20	92

TABLE 7.22
Month of Accident

Month	Number	Month	Number
January	0	July	36
February	0	August	20
March	1	September	2
April	2	October	2
May	8	November	0
June	21	December	0
		Total	92

of the accidents. Only six (6.5%) accidents occurred before noon, and seven (7.6%), from noon until 2 P.M.

MONTH OF ACCIDENT

The month in which the accidents occurred is shown in Table 7.22. As expected, 77(83.7%) of the accidents occurred during the summer months of June, July, and August.

YEAR OF ACCIDENT

Table 7.23 records the years in which the accidents occurred. The 92 accidents covered a 20-year period from pre-1970 through 1989. It is essential to understand that these are individual case studies and in no way represent all the springboard diving accidents that occurred in this time frame.

TABLE 7.23
Year of Accident

Year	Number	Year	Number
Before 1970	1	1980	6
1970	2	1981	7
1971	2	1982	6
1972	1	1983	9
1973	4	1984	6
1974	4	1985	6
1975	5	1986	4
1976	4	1987	3
1977	5	1988	4
1978	4	1989	4
1979	5	Total	92

TABLE 7.24
Victim's Visits to the Pool

Visits	First	Prior	Total
None	50	0	50
One or two	0	17	17
Three or more	0	25	25
Total	50	42	92

TABLE 7.25
Dives Made on Prior Visits

Dives	Number
None	23
One to three	2
Four or more	17
Total	42

Victim's Visits to the Pool

Tables 7.24 to 7.26 present data on the victim's familiarity with the pool. Table 7.24 indicates that in 50(54.3%) of the cases the victim was visiting the pool for the first time. This is a most significant fact when considering who is at greatest risk.

Dives Made on Previous Visits

Of the 42 victims who had been to the pool on previous occasions, 23(54.8%) had made no dives during those visits as shown in Table 7.25.

Dives Made on Day of Accident

Table 7.26 shows 50(54.3%) were injured on their first dive into the pool.

Type of Social Setting

In every instance the victim was a member of a social gathering, as shown in Table 7.27. An impromptu party or get-together accounted for 82(89.1%) of the events. In only ten (10.9%) instances was the victim attending a formal party, which had been previously planned with verbal or written invitations being given to guests.

Substance Abuse

Table 7.28 describes substance abuse. Only 3(3.3%) of the 92 victims admitted or were identified by others to have consumed any form of drugs on the day they were injured. However, it was

TABLE 7.26
Dives Made on Day of Accident

Dives	Number
First	50
Two to three	30
Four or more	12
Total	92

TABLE 7.27
Type of Social Setting

Setting	Number
Informal	82
Formal	10
Total	92

TABLE 7.28
Substance Abuse

Substance	Yes	No	Total
Alcohol	36	56	92
Drugs	3	89	92

TABLE 7.29
Posted Rules and Warning Signs

Instructions	Yes	No	Total
Posted rules	52	40	92
Warning signs	6	86	92

TABLE 7.30
Lifeguard on Duty

Lifeguard	Number
Yes	20
No	72
Total	92

established that drugs were present at or near the pool in seven (7.6%) of the cases. On the other hand, 36(39.1%) of the victims had consumed some form of alcoholic beverage (mostly beer) prior to the accident. The quantity ranged from one beer to more than four. Blood alcohol levels were taken in only four of the cases. The residential pool, usually involving a party, was the predominant scene where alcohol was consumed.

SAFETY AND SUPERVISION

Safety and supervision include the efforts of pool owners to provide posted instructions and warning signs.

POSTED RULES AND WARNING SIGNS

Table 7.29 shows the presence of posted rules and warning signs. Posted rules pertaining to the use of the pool were evident at 52(56.5%) of the accident sites. Most were of a general nature such as hours of operation, restriction against bringing in food or alcoholic beverages, no horseplay, no running, no scuba equipment, requirement that bathers shower before entering pool, etc. In 40(43.5%) cases there were no pool rules. None of the pools had rules that addressed diving safety.

Warning or caution signs pertaining to diving were present in only 6(6.5%) of the pools. In 86(93.5%) cases, victims did not have the benefit of posted instructions or warning signs concerning diving off the springboard or jumpboard.

LIFEGUARD ON DUTY

In 72(78.3%) of the cases there was no qualified lifeguard—paid or unpaid—on duty at the pool where the accident occurred, as shown in Table 7.30. The 20(21.7%) locations where supervision was present were invariably at public (city or county), school, or club pools.

RESCUE PROCEDURES

How the victims were rescued and who removed them from the pool after their injury were of great concern to the investigators. The chance of aggravating the injury to the spinal cord is very possible if proper procedures are not followed in the rescue attempt.

TABLE 7.31
Person Making Rescue

Rescuer	Number
Friends and other swimmers	70
Lifeguard	18
EMS	4
Total	92

TABLE 7.32
Use of Spineboard and CPR

Technique	Yes	No	Total
Spineboard	6	86	92
CPR	10	82	92

TABLE 7.33
Paramedics Involved

Paramedics	Number
Yes	82
No	10
Totals	92

Table 7.31 highlights the need for educating people as to the proper procedures to follow when a person is suspected of having a spinal injury.

PERSON MAKING RESCUE

Only 4(4.4%) of the 92 victims were removed from the water by a rescue squad or emergency medical services (EMS) using a spineboard. Lifeguards removed 18(19.6%), usually with the assistance of other swimmers. The majority (70, 76.1%) were removed by friends or other swimmers.

USE OF SPINEBOARD AND CARDIOPULMONARY RESUSCITATION

A disturbing fact, revealed in Table 7.32, shows that in only 6(6.5%) of the 92 cases was the victim removed from the water using a spineboard. This means that the vast majority were lifted, pulled, or dragged out of the water by friends who, in general, were not aware of the injury. This statistic clearly identifies the lack of knowledge of people concerning the identification of spinal cord victims and the proper techniques to be used in their removal from the water. Rescue breathing was employed in 10(10.9%) cases. This implies that the rescue of the victim was probably achieved within a minute or two from the time of injury.

PARAMEDIC INVOLVEMENT

Paramedics were used in all but 10(10.9%) of the 92 cases, as shown in Table 7.33, but few arrived in time to remove the victim from the water.

CONCLUSIONS

The data on springboard/jumpboard diving provided valuable information related to the circumstances surrounding these diving injuries. The conclusions set forth are not only drawn from the accumulated data but also from the research conducted by Gabrielsen and others. Considerable information was also obtained by the review of plans of the pool, the diving equipment involved, and the manner in which the pool was operated, the interviews with 86 of the victims, and the sworn testimony of victims and witnesses to the accident.

It is the hope of the authors that those responsible for the design and operation of pools as well as the manufacturers of springboard/jumpboards give careful consideration to the findings and recommendations contained in this book. Furthermore, we urge all governmental agencies responsible for developing laws and regulations governing the specifications for pools to study this book. Our conclusions are as follows:

POOLS WHERE THE ACCIDENT OCCURRED

Bottom Configuration

In 92 of the springboard/jumpboard accidents reported in this book, *the configuration of the bottom of the pool in the longitudinal axis was either a spoon or hopper shape.* In the spoon configuration, the maximum depth occurred at a single point, which was usually the location of the pool main drain. The upslope of the bottom (transition) leading up to the shallow end of the pool starts at that point. In the hopper bottom, the area of maximum depth varied in accordance with the size of the pool hopper. The length of the maximum depth area in the hopper-bottom pool ranged in size from 4 to 6 ft.

Depth of Water Where Victim Struck Bottom

Probably the most significant revelation was that *none of the divers when injured struck the bottom of the pool at the maximum water depth.* All the injured divers made contact with the bottom of the pool on the upslope, the transition between deep and shallow water. In several cases the diver completely overshot the designated deep water or diving area of the pool.

Type of Diving Equipment

Of the 38(44.6%) diving accidents that occurred in public pools, 23(29.7%) were of the competitive-type diving boards—either 14 or 16 ft long, and 15(13.8%) were 3-m-high springboards. One board was placed 2 m above the water. None of the pools involved in these accidents met the specifications promulgated by the following competitive diving groups: United States Diving (USD), National Collegiate Athletic Association (NCAA), International Swim and Dive Federation (FINA), and National Federation of State High School Athletic Associations (NFSHSAA).

The type of diving boards employed in the residential pools ranged from 6 to 10 ft in length for conventional-type springboards, while the jumpboards ranged in length from 3 to 8 ft. It is time to ask the following question: "Is it necessary to have the great variety in the lengths of boards and the dozen or more different mountings or stands and fulcrums?" It would appear that the time has come for some standardization in the design and placement of these recreational-type boards and stands.

Lack of Depth Markers

None of the 57 residential pools involved had any depth markers that would inform the diver as to the water depth in the diving area.

Lack of Posted Rules

Only 52(56.5%) of the 92 pools involved had any rules posted concerning the use of the diving board.

INDUSTRY STANDARDS AND GOVERNMENT REGULATIONS

Industry Standards are in Error

The standards pertaining to the geometric specifications of the pool diving envelope published by the National Spa and Pool Institute (NSPI) do not reflect the knowledge about divers' performance and equipment that has been generated by diving board studies and the experience of teachers and coaches. In our opinion, the NSPI's suggested standards for the pool diving area in both residential and public pools are in error and mislead pool builders.

NSPI Water Depth Unsafe

The maximum water depth recommended by NSPI is not safe for springboard diving by adults or teenagers of adult size.

Adults Should Not Dive into Residential Pools

Based on our findings, none of the residential pools in the study can safely accommodate diving from springboards or jumpboards by adults.

Excessive Variety of Boards and Stands

There is a proliferation of springboards/jumpboards and their attendant mountings that manufacturers have produced and made available to the builders, operators, and owners of pools. The board manufacturers have produced over 30 different types/models of springboards/jumpboards and stands. We do not believe that there is a need for this great a variety of boards and stands.

Transition Upslope Too Close to the End of the Springboard

The transition upslope between the deep and shallow portions of the pool was, in every instance, too close to the end of the springboard and was the defect that caused most of the injuries discussed in this book.

Hopper- and Spoon-Type Pools Unsafe for Diving

The hopper-bottom and spoon-shaped pools do not provide sufficient volume of water for safe diving, and the conclusion of the authors is that it is not safe to install springboards/jumpboards in these types of pools.

THE VICTIMS

Age and Sex

Of the 92 victims, 80(87.0%) were over the age of 15, and 54(58.7%) were over the age of 18. This explodes the myth that young teenagers are at greatest risk. The fact that 86(93.5%) of the victims were males supports the theory that males tend to be more aggressive than females and yield more readily to peer pressure.

Use of Alcoholic Beverages and Drugs

Of the 92 victims, 36(39.1%) had consumed some alcoholic beverage the day of the accident, but only 3(3.3%) were deemed to have been intoxicated; another 3(3.3%) of the victims admitted to the consumption of some form of drugs.

Diving Training

None of the victims had ever received any formal instruction in diving from a qualified teacher or coach. There appeared to be a marked inconsistency in the diving technique of the victims, which indicates that at times they had no control over their dives.

Appearance of Safety

It was evident that the victims misinterpreted the conditions that existed in the pool and its surrounding area. Some had seen other successful dives before they had dived. All thought that it was safe to dive and when asked the question, "Would you have dived if someone or a sign had warned you of the danger of diving into the pool?" Their unanimous response was "No!"

Victim: Guest or Owner

Most of the victims were guests of pool owners (homeowner or motel/hotel) or of tenants of apartments with pools. For 50(54.4%) of the victims, it was their first visit to the pool and they were injured on the first dive. The conclusion that can be drawn from this is that the owners of the pools were not communicating adequately with the victims concerning the rules of the pool and inherent dangers and hazards that existed if someone should dive into the pool.

SUMMARY

The data presented in this chapter makes it evident that the recommended design of pool diving envelopes by the NSPI for both residential and public pools needs to be corrected. See Chapter 12 for the recommendations of the authors for designs of the diving well in these types of pools.

8   Starting Block Diving Accidents

INTRODUCTION

This chapter contains the findings related to injuries that occurred as a result of individuals diving from starting blocks into inground swimming pools. A starting block is used by swimmers at the start of swimming races, as shown in Figure 8.1. Excluded from this study are dives made into inground pools from springboards and jumpboards, which are covered in Chapter 7.

We have investigated 32 injuries involving dives off starting blocks, using the same data form used in all other pool-rated diving cases. Once the data were collected, they were then computerized and various tables were developed and placed in the following categories:

- Victims
- Pool facilities
- Environmental factors
- Pre- and postaccident Events
- Safety and supervision
- Rescue procedures

SOME BACKGROUND ON THE PROBLEM

We consider it important to describe how these injuries occurred and why they occurred; consequently, we present the following history of the development of starting blocks.

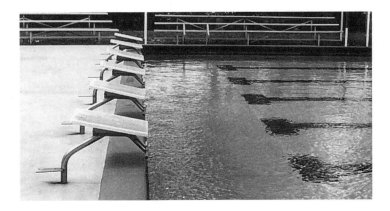

FIGURE 8.1 Typical 30-in.-high starting block.

Evolution of the Racing Start in Swimming

Period between the 1920s and 1930s

In the 1920 to 1930 era, swimming races were started from the edge of the deck of the pool, usually at a height of 8 to 10 in. above the water. There were only two exceptions. One was at Boys' Club pools, with the 1937 introduction of the "deck level" pool in which the gutter was incorporated into a trench located in the deck some 12 in. from the edge of the pool. The other exception was at YMCA pools, with the 1930 introduction of the "roll-out gutter," and the 1950 introduction of the "open gutter." It became apparent to those operating these pools that some kind of elevated platform was needed to achieve a proper racing entry.

During the 1920s and 1930s swimmers started races by placing their toes over the edge of the pool, and assuming a crouched position, with the arms extended behind the body. Coaches and swimmers then began experimenting with letting the arms hang vertically before the sound of the gun. Swimmers would then swing the arms back as they started their lean forward and would quickly pull them forward as they propelled the body from the blocks. The same arm positions were used when the blocks were introduced (Figure 8.2). Several other experiments followed relative to the position and action of the arms. One positioned the arms forward of the body followed by the swimmer rapidly swinging the arms in a circular motion. It proved to be of little help.

In the early period (1920 to 1940), as the swimmer left the pool deck he propelled the body forward, reaching out as far as possible and landing flat on the surface of the water (Figure 8.3). Hence, the dive was designated as a "flat racing dive," or as some have labeled it, the "conventional flat dive." Almost immediately on entry into the water, the swimmer after a short glide would then start the kick and arm stroke, whether freestyle, breaststroke, or butterfly (Figure 8.4).

Starting Blocks Approved in 1940

The same basic mechanics were used when the 18-in.-high starting blocks were approved for use in this country in 1940 by the ruling bodies for competitive swimming Amateur Athletic Union (AAU) and the National Collegiate Athletic Association (NCAA). The exact wording describing the start of swimming races in the 1940 NCAA Official Rules for Swimming, Fancy Diving, and Water Polo follow:

> Section 1. It is recommended that pools for championship meets shall be at least 75 feet in length and at least 35 feet in width, and have a water depth of at least ten feet in the deep end and not less than three feet in the shallow end, and the height of the take-off for all races shall be 18 inches above the surface of the water. The take-off must be flat and parallel to the surface of the water. It is further recommended that firm starting grips flush with the end of the pool be provided for backstroke swimming starts.

All collegiate, high school, YMCA, and Boys' Club facilities followed these rules. In 1954, the NCAA rules, which also governed scholastic swimming, added these options:

- The takeoff shall be a minimum of 18 in. and must not exceed 30 in. above the water. The takeoff must be parallel to the surface of the water.
- The reference to the flatness of the surface was subsequently removed from the rules in the 1971 NCAA rule book, with the takeoff to be sloped toward the pool not more than 10 degrees from the horizontal.

In the 1958 rules, the blocks were raised to a height of 0.75 m (30 in.). The new rule stated that starting blocks, 30 in. above the surface of the water should be provided for dual meets and must be provided for championship meets.

From the introduction of blocks in 1940 until 1970, the top surface of the blocks were level. In 1971, the rule was modified to permit the surface of the block to "slope toward the pool not

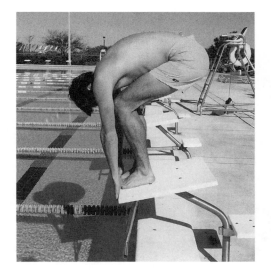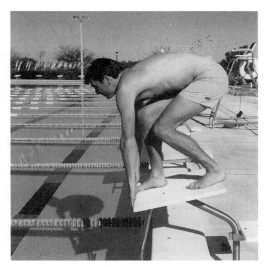

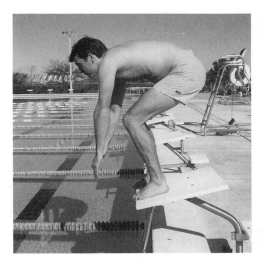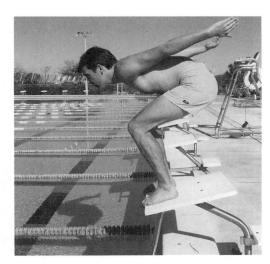

FIGURE 8.2 Variations of swimmer's arm position on starting blocks.

more than 10 degrees from the horizontal." This new rule pertaining to the height of the block signaled the end of the option of having the height of the block at 18 in. This change, in all probability, was intended to make the U.S. swimming rules consistent with the International Swim and Dive Federation (FINA) rules. Both the NCAA and AAU adopted this new rule.

Initially, after the increase in the height of the block, swimmers continued to employ the flat dive with arms in the positions described previously. However, it did not take the swimmers and their coaches very long to realize that when landing flat, the face and stomach received a pretty good smack and the forward momentum of the swimmer was impeded by the body's resistance to the water.

Increased Angle of Entry

Subsequently, the next step in the progression was for the swimmer to enter the water at a greater angle—about 15 to 20 degrees from the horizontal. The swimmer's entry into the water at this angle was not clean; therefore, some coaches began to experiment with entry angles of 25 to 30 degrees (Figure 8.5). This adjustment proved to be acceptable until swimmers introduced the use

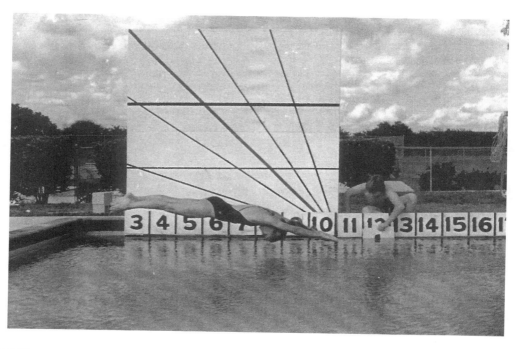

FIGURE 8.3 The flat racing dive.

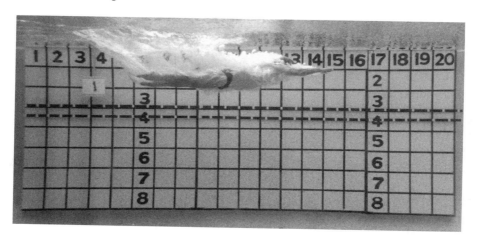

FIGURE 8.4 Underwater photo of diver making a shallow dive.

of goggles. This was done to enable them to better visualize the bottom line and turning target on the wall, thereby assisting them in swimming straighter and in the execution of their turns. Swimmers realized that it was almost impossible to keep the goggles in place when executing the flat or semiflat dive involving an entry angle up to 30 degrees. To have the goggles forced out of the eye socket by the force of water and hanging from the neck invariably meant the loss of the race. These phenomena became apparent probably in the late 1960s and early 1970s. The solution became readily obvious. Swimmers and coaches concluded that the entry must be at a steeper angle, with the head flexed in a near vertical position. This position would avoid water pressure directly on the goggles. However, one of the problems this move created was that the swimmer's entry point was reduced by as much as a foot, which in a tight race could mean the loss of the race.

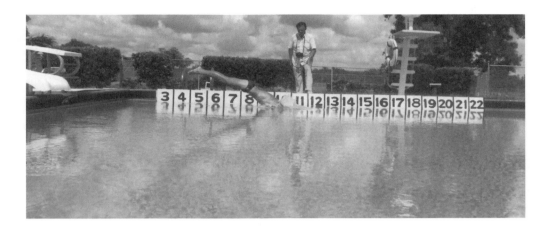

FIGURE 8.5 Swimmer employing a 25- to 30-degree angle of entry.

Introduction of the "Pike Dive"

About this time (1970s), coaches and swimmers throughout the country began to introduce a gymnastic movement at the height of the swimmer's dive that resulted in an entry angle between 40 and 50 degrees. In essence, this is what happens. After the takeoff from the blocks and as the swimmer reaches the height of his trajectory, he bends at the waist placing the body into a semijackknife position and then proceeds with a vigorous action to straighten the body as it starts the downward path and enters the water with the body fully aligned at an angle of about 45 degrees. The body is streamlined and follows the hands, arms, and head into the water in what has been described by some as a "clean entry." The higher the dive, the greater the entry speed.

This gymnastic movement received several names by coaches as it emerged onto the swimming scene. Some called it the "pike dive" and others described it as the "dive into the hole"; still others labeled it as the "scoop dive." It is interesting that each of these labels, in reality, describes a specific phase of the dive. The pike occurs during the body's movement through the air, the hole is the entry point, and the scoop describes the underwater path of the diver. (See Figure 8.6 for a comparison of the flat and pike dives.)

Grab Start

The "grab start" was first introduced by Hanauer[1] whereby the swimmer grips the front edge of the starting block with his hands, either between or outside the feet. One manufacturer of starting blocks placed handrails on the top surface of the block for swimmers to grab hold of. Counsilman[2] descibed the grab start as "at the sound of the gun, the swimmer pulls himself downward and forward, diving into the water with his body inclined at an angle of 15 to 30 degrees with the surface of the water and the hands and head lower than the feet." There is no question that the grab start provides the swimmer with greater stability while on the block, consequently resulting in fewer false starts. There is little supporting evidence, however, that it is faster than other starts, as suggested by Hanauer[3]. Lowell[4] also indicated that the grab start was faster.

No attempt has been made by the authors to determine what the swimmers in foreign countries were doing. However, Levin[5] in collaboration with others describes the racing start in his book titled *Swimming*. No mention is made of the pike dive. Levin and colleagues labeled the grab start as the "grip start." Their recommendation is that in the flight phase the body is kept extended from the fingertips to the toe tips as the swimmer "slips" into the water at an angle of about 20 to 25 degrees. No mention was made of the potential danger of swimmers striking the bottom.

Fitzgerald introduced a variation of the conventional method of placing both feet on the edge of the block in the 1970s. It involved the swimmers grabbing the front of the block with their hands and placing their feet in a position where one foot was on the front edge and the other was back, resembling the start used in track meets. This start was best performed from blocks having a 10-degree slope to the top of the block. However, this start required a modification of the rule permitting blocks to have a length of 36 in.

Counsilman[2] with others studied which of the three following starts was fastest: the flat, the track, or the scoop. The conclusion was that the flat entry was the fastest and the scoop, the slowest.

DANGERS ASSOCIATED WITH THE PIKE DIVE

The pike dive has been previously described, but the mechanics involved have not.

NEED FOR GREATER PRECISION

The pike dive must be executed with great precision when performed in shallow water or disaster may occur. There are two crucial phases of the dive. The first is the angle of the body as it enters the water. It must not exceed 45 degrees. The second is the need for the diver to plane and level off immediately on entry. An entry angle steeper than 45 degrees could cause the swimmer to go into a snap roll where the body rolls forward into a somersault. This is not very common, but it can happen.

NEED FOR IMMEDIATE PLANING

Immediately upon entry, the swimmer needs to try to achieve a body plane parallel to the surface at a depth of $2\frac{1}{2}$ to 3 ft. This is critical both to the success of the dive and to the prevention of possible contact with the bottom in pools with a depth of $3\frac{1}{2}$ ft. The diver has only 0.2 to 0.3 of a second to accomplish this planing. Therefore, the diver must be programmed in advance (know what he must do) to execute the movement. The action should be so automatic that the diver does not have to think about it. This is only achieved by practice, practice, practice. Figure 8.6 contains an excellent comparison between the flat and pike dive. The purpose of the pike dive, as explained previously, is to prevent the goggles from coming off. When the pike dive is executed in deep water, the diver may become careless and penetrate to a depth of 4 to 5 ft, which results in a loss of time.

In 1990, the National Federation of State High School Athletic Associations (NFSHSAA) was the first ruling body to do something about the question of starting blocks by making the following announcement:

IMPORTANT NOTICE

TO ALL HIGH SCHOOL COACHES & SWIMMERS

Due to three catastrophic injuries to competitive high school swimmers during the 1989–90 school year, the National Federation of State High School Athletic Associations' Swimming & Diving Rules Committee has noted the following revision: "In pools with water depth less than 4 ft. at the starting end, starting platforms shall be no more than 18" above the water surface or be located at the deep end of the pool."
This rule becomes effective with the 1991–92 season.

LIMIT YOUR RISK.

ALSO LET YOUR TEAM BECOME ACCUSTOMED

TO THIS NEW RACING HEIGHT NOW.

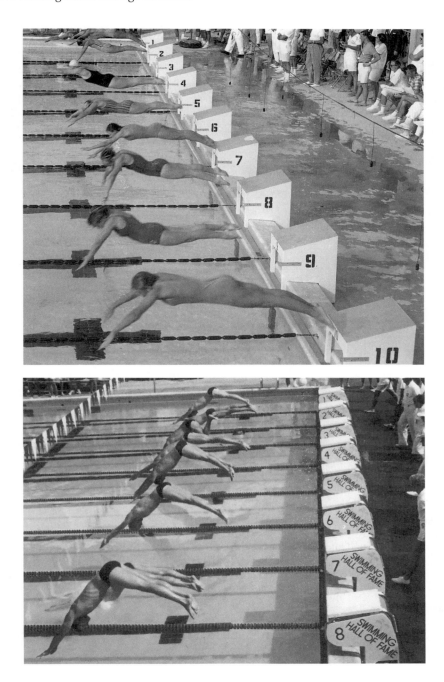

FIGURE 8.6 Top: the flat racing dive. Bottom: the pike dive used by divers at a national championship.

In our opinion, this notice falls short of what needs to be done and will not reduce the number of injuries occurring off starting blocks (Figure 8.7).

It is the hope of the authors that all those concerned with competitive swimming—coaches, pool administrators, governing bodies for competitive swimming, architects and engineers who design pools, and various regulatory agencies—will carefully consider the findings and recommendations contained in this book. The primary purpose of the publication is to provide aquatic professionals

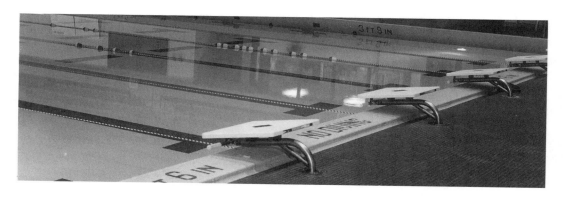

FIGURE 8.7 Blocks reduced to height of 18 in.

TABLE 8.1
Age and Sex of Victims

Age	Males	Females	Total
10–12	0	2	2
13–15	8	8	16
16–18	9	2	11
19–21	1	0	1
22–24	1	1	2
Total	19	13	32

and owners of pools with the information necessary for them to take positive action to eliminate these catastrophic injuries.

VICTIMS

AGE AND SEX

Table 8.1 indicates the age and sex of the victims. Only 2(6.3%) of the 32 were older than 21, and 1(3.1%) was a recreational swimmer making the first dive from a starting block during a physical education class. Of the 32 victims, 29(90.6%) were age 18 or below.

HEIGHT AND WEIGHT

Table 8.2 records the victims' height at the time of injury. Table 8.3 indicates the weight of the victims. Of the males 13(40.6%) weighed over 170 lb.

LEVEL OF INJURY

Table 8.4 indicates the level of spinal and other injuries, as revealed in the medical records.

SOURCE OF INITIAL SWIMMING AND DIVING INSTRUCTION

Table 8.5 indicates that 28(87.5%) of the individuals learned to swim by the time they were 8 years old.

Table 8.6 reveals that self-instruction or instruction by parent or family was the source of initial diving instruction for 24(75.0%) of the victims.

TABLE 8.2
Height of Victims

Height (ft/in.)	Males	Females	Total
5/0	0	2	2
5/1	0	0	0
5/2	0	2	2
5/3	0	1	1
5/4	0	4	4
5/5	1	1	2
5/6	0	1	1
5/7	2	1	3
5/8	0	1	1
5/9	1	0	1
5/10	6	0	6
5/11	2	0	2
6/0	3	0	3
6/1	0	0	0
6/2	2	0	2
6/3	0	0	0
6/4	1	0	1
6/5	1	0	1
Total	19	13	32

TABLE 8.3
Weight of Victims

Weight (lb)	Males	Females	Total
90–99	0	1	1
100–109	0	4	4
110–119	0	2	2
120–129	0	3	3
130–139	1	0	1
140–149	2	0	2
150–159	2	0	2
160–169	1	1	2
170–179	6	0	6
180–189	4	1	5
190–199	0	0	0
200–209	0	0	0
210–219	0	0	0
220–229	0	0	0
230–239	2	0	2
240–249	1	1	2
Total	19	13	32

TABLE 8.4
Level of Injury

Level	Males	Females	Total
C-4	3	0	3
C-4, 5	6	2	8
C-5	4	3	7
C-5, 6	5	5	10
C-6	1	0	1
C-6, 7	0	2	2
Fractured arm and concussion	0	1	1
Total	19	13	32

TABLE 8.5
Age Victim Learned to Swim

Age	Number
1–4	6
5–8	22
9–12	3
13 and over	1
Total	32

TABLE 8.6
Source of Initial Diving Instruction

Source	Number
Self-taught	10
Parent or family member	14
City recreation department	2
American Red Cross	3
School or college	2
YMCA	1
Total	32

TABLE 8.7
Pool Ownership

Owner	Number
High school/college	22
Municipality (city/county)	5
Voluntary agency	4
Other (U.S. Navy)	1
Total	32

POOL FACILITIES

The following tables present specifications and other characteristics of the pools where the starting black accidents occurred.

POOL OWNERSHIP

Table 8.7 identifies the owner of the pool where the accident occurred. High schools or colleges were the location of 22(68.8%) of the accidents.

LOCATION BY STATE

There were 15 different states where these accidents occurred with five (15.6%) in Illinois, four (12.5%) in California and Pennsylvania, and three (9.4%) in Ohio (as shown in Table 8.8).

POOL SHAPES

Table 8.9 identifies the various shapes of the pools involved. Most were rectangular in shape with both a shallow and deep end.

BASIN COMPOSITION

Table 8.10 identifies the pool basin composition. All the accident pools had a poured concrete basin.

TABLE 8.8
Location by State

State	Number
Illinois	5
California	4
Pennsylvania	4
Ohio	3
New York	2
Indiana	2
Michigan	2
Wisconsin	2
Wyoming	2
Alabama	1
Colorado	1
Florida	1
Kansas	1
Massachusetts	1
North Carolina	1
Total	32

TABLE 8.9
Pool Shapes

Shape	Number
Conventional, rectangular	27
"T"	3
"L"	2
Total	32

Basin Composition**

Finish	Number
Poured concrete	32
Total	32

**TABLE 8.11
Pool Markings**

Marking	Yes	No	Total
Depth markings	32	0	32
Bottom markings	0	32	32
Lifeline in place	0	32	32

**TABLE 8.12
Clarity of Water**

Clarity	Number
Empty	0
Clear	30
Semiturbid	2
Turbid	0
Total	32

**TABLE 8.13
Lighting and Weather**

Factor	Yes	No	Total
Lighting	0	32	32
Weather	0	32	32

POOL MARKINGS

Table 8.11 indicates that all the pools had depth markings while none had bottom markings. Lifelines were absent in each case because of the accidents occurred during swim meets or practices.

ENVIRONMENTAL FACTORS

CLARITY OF WATER

In all but two (6.3%) of the accident sites, the pool water was clear (Table 8.12).

LIGHTING AND WEATHER

Table 8.13 presents two environmental factors, namely, lighting and weather. Lighting, that is illumination in and around the pool, was adequate in every case; and weather was not a factor because all sites were indoors.

PRE- AND POSTACCIDENT EVENTS

This section covers the elements related to the pre- and postaccident events, as well as the circumstances directly related to the accident and a description of the specific activity involved.

WHEN ACCIDENT OCCURRED

Table 8.14 identifies the nature of the activity the victim engaged in when the accident occurred. Only two (6.3%) actually occurred at the start of a race.

DESCRIPTION OF TYPE OF DIVE

Table 8.15 identifies the type of dive the victim performed that resulted in the injury. Pike dives were performed in 19(59.4%) instances with 4(12.5%) involving the use of an instructional aid (1 using rubber tubing, 2 using a rope, and 1 diving through a hula hoop).

The remaining 13(40.6%) injuries included 4(12.5%) ordinary front dives performed by recreational divers, not members of a swim team; the 3(9.4%) injuries that involved loss of balance were false starts with the exception of one indicating loss of balance because of an unstable starting block. The vault was more or less a stunt suggested by the coach whereby the swimmer placed the hands on the top platform of the block and pushed off with the body going forward into a dive. The diver apparently failed to maintain a body position parallel to the water. According to witnesses, the diver's upper torso was bent at the trunk causing water entry at a critical angle. The somersault false start is a no, no. All swimmers must be instructed to make a regular dive instead of rolling forward into a somersault during a false start.

INSTRUCTIONS TO SWIMMERS RELATIVE TO PIKE DIVE

Of the 19 dives involving the pike position, only 12(63.2%) of the victims had received any instruction from the coach concerning the mechanics of the start; and victims indicated that no emphasis was placed on the potential danger of striking the bottom if the dive was improperly executed. Furthermore, there was no evidence of any type of lead-up activities such as starting dives first from blocks placed at the deep end of the pool.

DEPTH OF WATER WHERE VICTIM STRUCK BOTTOM

In every one of the 32 cases, the estimated depth of water where the victim made contact with the bottom was 4 ft or less. Most of the pools involved had a depth at the starting block of $3\frac{1}{2}$ feet, which then gradually started to slope down, and consequently the water would be slightly deeper at the point of impact with the bottom.

TABLE 8.14
When Accident Occurred

Activity	Number
During regular practice session	17
During recreational swim period	6
During warm-up before meet	6
At start of a race	2
During regular P.E. class	1
Total	32

TABLE 8.15
Description of Type of Dive

Dive	Number
Pike dive	19
Regular with no aids (14)	
With aids (4)	
With swim fins (1)	
Ordinary front dive (no pike) 30-degree entry	4
Lost balance or slipped on block	3
Flat dive 15- to 20-degree entry	4
Vault off block	1
False start (somersault)	1
Total	32

Member of Swim Team

Victims were members of a swim team in 28(87.5%) of the cases, as shown in Table 8.16; the other 4(12.5%) were recreational swimmers who were just trying out the starting blocks because they had seen others do it.

Swim Coach Present

In every one of the 28 cases involving a swim team member, the team coach or assistant was present.

Victim: Guest or Pool Owner

Table 8.17 addresses the issue of whether the victim was a guest or the owner.

Time and Day of Accident

As Table 8.18 indicates, 28(87.5%) of the accidents occurred between the hours of 2 and 6 P.M. The injuries all occurred on Thursday, Friday, or Saturday.

Month of Accident

Table 8.19 indicates the month in which the injury to the victim occurred.

TABLE 8.16
Member of Swim Team

Team	Number
High school	22
Junior high school	5
College	1
No team (recreational swimmer)	4
Total	32

TABLE 8.17
Victim: Guest or Owner

Victim	Number
Guest	32
Owner	0
Total	32

TABLE 8.18
Time and Day of Accident

Time Interval	Mon.	Tue.	Wed.	Thu.	Fri.	Sat.	Sun.	Total
12:00–01:59 A.M.	0	0	0	0	0	0	0	0
02:00–03:59 A.M.	0	0	0	0	0	0	0	0
04:00–05:59 A.M.	0	0	0	0	0	0	0	0
06:00–07:59 A.M.	0	0	0	0	0	0	0	0
08:00–09:59 A.M.	0	0	0	0	0	0	0	0
10:00–11:59 A.M.	0	0	0	0	0	0	0	0
12:00–01:59 P.M.	0	0	0	0	0	0	0	0
02:00–03:59 P.M.	0	0	0	2	10	4	0	16
04:00–05:59 P.M.	0	0	0	0	6	6	0	12
06:00–07:59 P.M.	0	0	0	2	0	0	0	2
08:00–09:59 P.M.	0	0	0	2	0	0	0	2
10:00–11:59 P.M.	0	0	0	0	0	0	0	0
Total	0	0	0	6	16	10	0	32

TABLE 8.19
Month of Accident

Month	Number
January	6
February	5
March	2
April	0
May	0
June	0
July	0
August	0
September	2
October	6
November	6
December	5
Total	32

TABLE 8.20
Year of Accident

Year	Number
1976	1
1977	2
1978	1
1979	1
1980	0
1981	2
1982	2
1983	3
1984	4
1985	1
1986	1
1987	3
1988	6
1989	4
1990	0
1991	1
Total	32

TABLE 8.21
Victim's Visits to the Pool

Visits	First	Prior	Total
None	12	0	12
One or two	0	5	5
Three or more	0	15	15
Total	12	20	32

TABLE 8.22
Dives made on Prior Visits

Dives	Number
None	0
One to three	10
Four or more	10
Total	20

YEAR OF ACCIDENT

Table 8.20 gives the year in which the accident happened. The years span from 1976 to 1991.

VICTIM'S VISITS TO THE POOL

Table 8.21 indicates that 12(37.5%) of the victims were visiting the pool for the first time, and 15 (46.9%) had previously been there three or more times.

DIVES MADE ON PRIOR VISITS

Of the 20 individuals who had visited the accident site previously, all had made at least one previous dive (Table 8.22).

DIVES MADE ON DAY OF ACCIDENT

Table 8.23 shows 8(25.0%) of the 32 victims were injured on their first dive into the pool.

TABLE 8.23
Dives Made on Day of Accident

Dives	Number
First	8
Two or three	10
Four or more	14
Total	32

TABLE 8.24
Type of Social Setting

Setting	Number
Informal	2
Formal/swim meet	30
Total	32

TABLE 8.25
Substance Abuse

Substance	Yes	No	Total
Alcohol	0	32	32
Drugs	0	32	32

TABLE 8.26
Posted Rules and Warning Signs

Instructions	Yes	No	Total
Posted rules	32	0	32
Warning signs	32	0	32

TABLE 8.27
Lifeguard on Duty

Lifeguard	Number
Yes	32
No	0
Total	32

TYPE OF SOCIAL SETTING

In every instance but two the setting was a swim meet. Two were recreational swimmers and not members of any swim team (Table 8.24).

SUBSTANCE ABUSE

As shown in Table 8.25, alcohol or drugs had not been consumed by any of the victims on the day of the accident.

WARNINGS AND SUPERVISION

POSTED RULES AND WARNING SIGNS

Pool rules and warning signs were present in all the pools, as shown in Table 8.26.

LIFEGUARD ON DUTY

In all these cases, the coach served as a lifeguard, as shown in Table 8.27.

TABLE 8.28 Person Making Rescue	
Rescuer	Number
Friends	1
Lifeguard	21
EMS	10
Total	32

TABLE 8.29 Use of Spineboard and CPR			
Technique	Yes	No	Total
Spineboard	32	0	32
CPR	10	22	32

RESCUE PROCEDURES

There is a need to educate individuals as to the proper procedures to follow when a person is suspected of having a spinal injury.

PERSON MAKING RESCUE

Table 8.28 identifies the person who made the initial rescue of the victim from the pool. The coach/ lifeguard made the majority of the rescues.

USE OF SPINEBOARD AND CARDIOPULMONARY RESUSCITATION

In all cases, the victim was removed from the water using a spineboard. This statistic clearly indicates that coaches were well informed concerning the identification of spinal cord victims and the proper techniques to be used in their removal. Rescue breathing, or cardiopulmonary resuscitation (CPR), was employed in ten (31.3%) cases. This implies that the rescue of the victim was probably achieved within a minute or two of the time of injury (Table 8.29).

CONCLUSIONS

After studying the 32 injuries resulting from dives off starting blocks, it became very clear why these injuries occurred. Our conclusions are as follows:

1. In every case, the shallowness of the water where the starting blocks were placed was the major cause of these accidents. Most of the depths in front of the blocks were $3\frac{1}{2}$ ft.
2. In only 1(3.1%) of the 32 cases was the swimmer a member of a college swim team.
3. Most of the high school and junior high school swimmers were beginners and had not received acceptable instructions as to the proper execution of the starts from their coaches.
4. We concluded that most of the coaches involved had failed to recognize the potential danger associated with diving off of a 30-in.-high starting block into $3\frac{1}{2}$ or 4 ft of water.
5. The coaches failed to adequately discuss with their swimmers the mechanics of the start and the potential danger of an improper start.
6. It was apparent that most of the injuries occurred when the victim was attempting to execute the pike dive.
7. We believe that the televising of national swimming meets depicting swimmers employing the pike dive start prompted young swimmers to emulate these experienced swimmers.
8. The ruling bodies of competitive swimming (NCAA, USS, and NFSHSAA) failed to act promptly to change their specifications for starting blocks with respect to the height of the block and depth of water.
9. We believe that if the depth of water where blocks are located is less than 5 ft, the blocks should be relocated to the deep end of the pool.

10. State regulatory agencies need to review their laws and regulations for public swimming pools in accordance with what we have recommended.
11. The reducing of the heights of the blocks to 18 in. is not feasible, in our opinion, unless the water depth is $4\frac{1}{2}$ ft.

REFERENCES

1. Hanauer, E. S., The grab start, *Swimming World*, No. 8, 1967.
2. Counsilman, J., Takeo, M., Motchin, E., and Counsilman, B., A Study of Three Types of Swimming Racing Starts, done by contract with the National Swimming Foundation, 1985.
3. Hanauer, E. S., Grab start faster than conventional start, *Swimming World*, No. 13, 1972.
4. Lowell, J., Analysis of the grab and conventional start, *Swimming Technique*, 13, No. 2, 1975.
5. Levin, G., *Swimming*, Sportverlag, Berlin, 1979.

9 Diving Accidents Occurring in the Natural Environment

INTRODUCTION

Of the 20,000 injuries from diving, 10,000 (50.0%) are the result of people diving into water bodies located in the natural environment. These are the lakes, rivers, oceans, ponds, embayments, reservoirs, ponds, quarries, and other water areas.

Natural water bodies represent the interaction of many dynamic forces—rain, drainage runoff, sedimentation, wind and waves, currents, floods, and ice jams. As a water body is changed by the upland or direct effects of man, many of the interactions are affected. Many philosophers of site planning believe that the first consideration of water-related planning is to leave the natural conditions undisturbed and build up to and around them. The edges or banks of water bodies such as streams, lakes, and rivers have been created by nature and often result in sandy beaches, bluffs, grass slopes, shrub entanglements, or tree roots that stabilize soil and control the on- and offshore water actions. All the dynamic forces at work must be clearly understood and either safely incorporated into the design and construction plans and subsequent supervision and operation of the area, or protected against in the development and management process.

Artificial water bodies also present a similar concern, particularly when they are altered by man for boating or drainage canals, storm water basins, drainage reservoirs or flood control channels, causeways, water storage basins, culvert settlement basins, and other structures, which present hazardous conditions or situations. From the smallest structure, its height of structure, depth and flow of water, surges, and washout all create serious problems for a person misusing such facilities. These natural bodies can result in entrapments, spearings, entanglements, and contusions, producing drowning or near drowning, brain injury, or quadriplegia.

BACKGROUND

Paralleling the post-World War II growth of pools has been the development of swimming beaches located along the shorelines of oceans, lakes, and rivers. Automotive transportation—not only cars but also campers, trailers, and motor homes—has placed previously inaccessible recreation areas within the reach of most people in the United States. National Parks, Forest Service land, as well as state and county parks, contain millions of acres of land, most of which contain lakes and rivers. Then there are the National and State Seashore Parks along the Atlantic and Pacific Oceans, the Great Lakes, the Gulfs, and other estuaries.

There are few designated swimming beaches in these areas. Therefore, it is not uncommon for vacationers en route to a campground or recreation park to stop and take a swim, which, in many instances, is in a nondesignated swimming area. Over 70 million visits are made to our National Parks each summer. Many vehicles driven to these vacation spots pull boats on trailers or carry rubber rafts, canoes, and a variety of small boats on the tops of their cars. Some bring with them fishing rods and reels, scuba diving gear, snorkeling equipment, surfboards, and water skis. For those who do not own such equipment, it is often available to rent when they arrive. Other water-related equipment (such as rowboats, sailboats, outboard motors, Hobie cats, windsurfers, and even kite flying over water pulled by a speedboat) is often also available on a rental basis at public and commercial beaches. In most cases rental equipment is operated by concessionaires on contract with a public agency or motel/hotel.

OWNERSHIP OF WATER AND SHORELINE PROPERTIES

Every body of water as well as the adjoining shoreline in the United States is owned by someone. Ownership of property and the adjoining water areas falls under different categories. To illustrate this, the following are listed. It should not be concluded that all agencies or individuals involved in ownership of land and water are identified.

FEDERAL GOVERNMENT

National Parks
U.S. Forest Service
Department of the Interior
Corps of Engineers
Tennessee Valley Authority
Department of Defense
Bureau of Land Management
Fish and Wildlife Service

STATE GOVERNMENTS

State parks and recreation areas
Water management departments
Reservoirs
Canals
Colleges and universities

COUNTY GOVERNMENTS

County parks and recreation areas
Water management departments
Reservoirs
Canals
Colleges and universities

CITY GOVERNMENTS

City parks and recreation areas
Reservoirs
Canals
Schools
Colleges and universities

PRIVATE ORGANIZATIONS

Schools, colleges, and universities
Girl and Boy Scouts

YMCA/YWCA
Fraternal organizations
Churches
Country clubs
Private individuals and organizations
Homeowners
Owners of vacation cottages
Farmers
Estate owners
Land developers and speculators
Homeowners' associations
Motels, hotels, and resorts
Industrial plants and mills
Utility owners
Children's camps
Campgrounds
Boat marinas
Mining companies
Logging companies
Hunting and fishing lodges
Commercially operated beaches

Before the Bureau of Outdoor Recreation was formed, it was estimated that 85% of the shoreline along the Atlantic coast was privately owned. A gradual decrease of private ownership has occurred as a result of the acquisition of property by various federal, state, and local governments made possible by federal grant programs and local bond issues.

When it comes to the nation's inland lakes and rivers, ownership ranges from federal, state, county, and local governments to private individuals, corporations, and groups. Most states provide public access to lakes or rivers by establishing easements. To a large extent, ownership of the land on the shorelines of lakes and rivers is by private individuals, many who build either permanent or vacation homes on their property. Also attracted to the acquisition of shoreline properties are resorts, campgrounds, children's camps, commercially operated boat marinas, and swimming beaches. Few rivers or lakes are owned by individuals. Most are owned by some governmental entity.

There are some interesting variations in ownership and leasing of property. For example, some private agencies owning a lake or reservoir have leased the use of the water to groups such as homeowners' associations for recreational activities such as boating, fishing, and swimming. In other instances, a federal or state agency may lease land on contract with a private individual or firm to operate facilities such as a swimming beach, fishing pier, or boat marina on a concession basis.

LACK OF PUBLIC AWARENESS

With the increasing participation of people in aquatic activities, it is inevitable that both diving and drowning accidents occur. Yet our study of 161 diving injuries reported in this chapter revealed that many of the accidents could have been prevented. The low level of public appreciation and under- standing of the hazards and risks inherent in many of the aquatic activities greatly increases the responsibility of everyone connected with the design and operation of these facilities. The education of the public to recognize hazards and exercise care when engaged in aquatic activities in unsupervised water areas is a challenge to both professional aquatic groups and governmental agencies.

If an impact is to be made on reducing the number of drowning and diving injuries occurring in the natural environment, it will require the combined efforts of governmental agencies, profes- sional organizations, aquatic professionals, and individual owners of water recreation areas.

Data derived from the sources indicated in Chapter 3 were recorded on a four-page collection form. Then the data were computerized, and various tables were developed and placed in the following categories:

- Victims
- Facilities
- Environmental Factors
- Pre- and Postaccident Events
- Safety and Supervision
- Rescue Procedures

This study did not address the question of the annual incidence of diving injuries occurring in the natural environment, or the relationship of these accidents to those occurring in pools. Furthermore, no attempt was made to determine the negligence of any of the parties involved or to record the outcome of lawsuits. The conclusions drawn from this study are exclusively those of the Editorial Board.

VICTIMS

AGE AND SEX

Table 9.1 shows the age and sex of the victims. Males represented 148 (91.9%) of the victims. Several interesting facts emerge. Males in the 19 to 21 year age category produced the most victims. The age bracket 16 to 24 represented 107 (72.3%) of the male victims. Of particular significance is that none was below the age of 13.

HEIGHT AND WEIGHT

Table 9.2 indicates that 102 (68.9%) of the males were 5 ft 10 in. or over. By contrast, females were more frequently 5 ft 6 in. or under.

Table 9.3 indicates that 79 males (53.4%) weighed 170 lb or more. The females typically weighed 130 lb or less.

TABLE 9.1
Age and Sex of Victims

Age	Males	Females	Total
13–15	13	0	13
16–18	40	2	42
19–21	44	6	50
22–24	23	2	25
25–27	8	1	9
28–30	8	1	9
31–33	8	0	8
34–36	2	1	3
37–39	1	0	1
40+	1	0	1
Total	148	13	161

TABLE 9.2
Height of Victims

Height (ft/in.)	Males	Females	Total
5/3	1	0	1
5/4	1	1	2
5/5	1	4	5
5/6	2	7	9
5/7	7	1	8
5/8	17	0	17
5/9	17	0	17
5/10	30	0	30
5/11	28	0	28
6/0	35	0	35
6/1	5	0	5
6/2	4	0	4
Total	148	13	161

TABLE 9.3
Weight of Victims

Weight (lb)	Males	Females	Total
110–119	2	5	7
120–129	3	5	8
130–139	7	2	9
140–149	15	1	16
150–159	15	0	15
160–169	27	0	27
170–179	49	0	49
180–189	15	0	15
190–199	8	0	8
200–209	3	0	3
210–219	2	0	2
220–229	1	0	1
230–239	1	0	1
Total	148	13	161

TABLE 9.4
Formal Diving Instruction

Instruction	Males	Females	Total
Self-taught	118	11	129
Some	30	2	32
Total	148	13	161

FORMAL DIVING INSTRUCTION

Formal diving instruction, as shown in Table 9.4, is based on participating in classes conducted by schools, the American Red Cross (ARC), or other agencies, as well as taking private lessons. As the figure illustrates, only 32(19.9%) of the victims had any formalized training in diving.

With respect to the diving skill level of the victims, there was no way to accurately determine this without having observed the dive or tested the victims. However, on the basis of the victim's own judgment of his ability as revealed in depositions and testimonies of family members and witnesses who were deposed, the conclusion was that all fell in the category of a recreational diver. Recreational divers are those individuals who never received training by a qualified diving coach.

LEVEL OF INJURY

Table 9.5 presents the level of the injuries to the spine. The range from C-4, 5 to C-5, 6 represented 122(75.8%) of the total injuries.

In summary, individuals at greatest risk are males, either adults or teenagers of adult size who have had no formal diving instruction.

FACILITIES

OWNERSHIP

Table 9.6 identifies the owner of the property or facility where the accident occurred. Corporations, such as motels and resort hotels, and commercially operated beaches or campgrounds owned 52 (32.3%) of the properties where the accidents occurred. The private ownership mostly involved vacation homes on lakes that usually had a dock extending out into the lake.

TABLE 9.5
Level of Injury

Level	Males	Females	Total
C-1	1	0	1
C-2, 3	1	0	1
C-3	1	0	1
C-4	1	2	3
C-4, 5	7	2	9
C-5	53	3	56
C-5, 6	54	3	57
C-6	8	0	8
C-6, 7	15	1	16
C-7	3	0	3
T-1, 2	0	1	1
T-3	1	0	1
Some neurological impairment	2	1	3
Paraplegia	1	0	1
Total	148	13	161

TABLE 9.6
Property Ownership

Owner	Number
Community/corporation	52
City	27
Private	29
State	16
U.S. government	13
County	12
Partnership	4
Church	3
University	2
Tenants' association	2
Utility	1
Total	161

TABLE 9.7
Site of Dive

Site	Number
Lake	90
River	32
Ocean	19
Pond	6
Quarry	1
Ocean embayment	7
Canal	4
Borrow pit	1
Intracoastal	1
Total	161

SITE OF DIVE

Table 9.7 reveals inland lakes accounted for 90(55.9%) of the accidents while 32(19.9%) happened in rivers. These two sites combined for over three quarters of the injuries.

LOCATION BY STATE

Table 9.8 indicates the state where the accident happened; as expected, Florida and California represented 60(37.3%) of the cases.

DESIGNATED SWIMMING AREA

As shown in Table 9.9, nearly half of the locations where accidents occurred were designated swimming areas. It was surprising in light of general opinion that the vast majority of accidents occur in unattended bodies of water.

TABLE 9.8
Location by State

State	Number	State	Number
Florida	42	Kansas	2
California	18	Kentucky	2
Michigan	12	Maryland	2
Illinois	9	Mississippi	2
Ohio	9	Nebraska	2
Arizona	8	New Jersey	2
Texas	7	Oklahoma	2
New York	7	South Carolina	2
North Dakota	5	Virginia	1
Arkansas	4	Wisconsin	1
Georgia	4	Colorado	1
Iowa	4	Delaware	1
Louisiana	4	Washington	1
Minnesota	4	Cayman Islands	1
Indiana	2	Total	161

TABLE 9.9
Designated Swimming Area

Designated Area	Number
Yes	74
No	87
Total	161

DEPTH OF WATER AT IMPACT

The data relative to the estimated depth of water where the victim struck the bottom, as shown in Table 9.10, were derived from statements of witnesses. The findings present a disturbing picture. In 26(16.1%) of the accidents the impact depth was 2 ft or less. In 137(85.1%) of the accidents the water was 4 ft deep or less.

ENVIRONMENTAL FACTORS

CLARITY OF WATER

Table 9.11 reveals that in only 11(6.8%) cases was the water at the accident site clear enough for the victim to see the bottom. Water was classified as turbid (muddy) in 131(81.4%) sites and semiturbid in 19(11.8%) sites. Interviews with victims and accounts of eye witnesses revealed that the bottom was not visible to the diver. This finding indicates that what we have been preaching for years, "know what you are diving into before you dive," has not reached everyone. Yet there was not a single victim who thought it was dangerous to dive where he did.

LIGHTING AND WEATHER

Lighting was a factor in only 15(9.3%) of the accidents, as shown in Table 9.12. In these instances, according to eyewitnesses, lighting was poor. Weather was even less likely to be a factor, having been mentioned in only 6(3.7%) of the 161 cases.

TABLE 9.10
Depth of Water at Impact

Depth (ft/in.)	Number
Not applicable	2
0/0	2
0/6	1
0/7–1/0	2
1/1–1/6	9
1/7–2/0	10
2/1–2/6	18
2/7–3/0	39
3/1–3/6	28
3/7–4/0	26
4/1–4/6	14
4/7–5/0	4
5/1–5/6	2
5/7–6/0	3
10/0	1
Total	161

TABLE 9.11
Clarity of Water

Clarity	Number
Turbid	131
Semiturbid	19
Clear	11
Total	161

TABLE 9.12
Lighting and Weather

Factor	Yes	No	Total
Lighting	15	146	161
Weather	6	155	161

PRE- AND POSTACCIDENT EVENTS

This section covers the elements related to the pre- and postaccident events, as well as the circumstances directly related to the accident and a description of the specific activity involved.

TIME AND DAY OF ACCIDENT

Table 9.13 reflects the time of day that the accident occurred. The P.M. hours represented 144(89.4%) of the accidents with noon to 6:00 P.M. representing 129(80.1%). Weekends represented the greatest likelihood that an accident would occur, with 90(55.9%) accidents occurring on Saturday and Sunday, as shown in Table 9.14.

MONTH OF ACCIDENT

Table 9.15 highlights that 114(70.8%) of the accidents happened, as expected, in the three summer months: June, July, and August.

YEAR OF ACCIDENT

Table 9.16 summarizes the years in which accidents occurred.

TABLE 9.13
Time of Day of Accident

12:00–01:59 A.M.	6
02:00–03:59 A.M.	1
04:00–05:59 A.M.	0
06:00–07:59 A.M.	0
08:00–09:59 A.M.	2
10:00–11:59 A.M.	8
12:00–01:59 P.M..	34
02:00–03:59 P.M.	55
04:00–05:59 P.M.	40
06:00–07:59 P.M.	13
08:00–09:59 P.M.	1
10:00–11:59 P.M.	1
Total	161

TABLE 9.14
Day of Week of Accident

Day	Number
Monday	14
Tuesday	7
Wednesday	13
Thursday	16
Friday	21
Saturday	40
Sunday	50
Total	161

TABLE 9.15
Month of Accident

Month	Number
January	1
February	2
March	4
April	6
May	26
June	30
July	54
August	30
September	4
October	2
November	2
December	0
Total	161

VICTIM'S VISITS TO THE SITE

Table 9.17 shows that 109(67.7%) of the injuries occurred on the victim's first visit to the site. An important finding from these data focuses on the risk involved for first-time visitors to an aquatic facility.

DIVES MADE ON DAY OF ACCIDENT

Table 9.18 presents data on the number of dives the victim made on the day of the accident. Most injuries—130(80.7%)—happened on the first dive.

POSITION OF ARMS/HANDS AT ENTRY

Table 9.19 reports witnesses' and victims' judgments on the position of the arms and hands during the dive that produced the injury. Hands were in front 150(93.2%) times.

TABLE 9.16
Year of Accident

Year	Number	Year	Number
1970	1	1985	9
1971	0	1986	9
1972	0	1987	8
1973	0	1988	3
1974	3	1989	5
1975	3	1990	1
1976	4	1991	1
1977	9	1992	2
1978	10	1993	2
1979	14	1994	4
1980	17	1995	2
1981	12	1996	3
1982	13	1997	2
1983	12	1998	2
1984	10	Total	161

TABLE 9.17
Victim's Visits to the Site

Visits	First	Prior	Total
None	109	0	109
One or two	0	22	22
Three or more	0	30	30
Total	109	52	161

TABLE 9.18
Dives Made on Day of Accident

Dives	Number
First	130
Two to three	20
Four or more	11
Total	161

TABLE 9.19
Position of Arms/Hands at Entry

Position	Number
In front	150
In between	8
At side	3
Total	161

LOCATION AND ACTIVITY

There were 23 different locations where the dive occurred as shown in Table 9.20. Diving from docks or piers into a lake or ocean accounted for the largest number (46, 28.6%) of the accidents while 30(18.6%) were dives from banks of rivers and lakes. Of the 21 dives made by victims running into the water and launching themselves into a dive, most occurred at designated swimming areas.

Of particular interest to the authors was that only 1(0.6%) of the 161 injuries was the result of the individual making a running dive into the ocean surf. One possible answer is that our public ocean beaches are well managed or that people who are injured in surf diving are reluctant to sue

TABLE 9.20
Location of Accident and Activity

Location and Activity	Number
Docks or piers into lake/ocean	46
Bank of river/lake	30
Run into river/lake	21
Retaining wall or bulkhead	16
Rope swing	7
Water slide	6
Bank or ledge of quarry	4
Boat	4
Bridge into river/lake	4
Branch of tree	3
Motel balcony/rooftop	3
Dive from cliff	3
Springboard	2
Dive from 10-m tower	2
Dive from jetty	2
Dive from 10-ft tower/hit swimmer in water	1
Dive from fountain into middle of pond	1
Run and dive into ocean surf	1
Dive from picnic table into river	1
Dive from water ski	1
Dive from top of water slide	1
Dive from drain pipe into lake	1
Thrown into lake	1
Total	161

TABLE 9.21
Substance Abuse

Substance	Yes	No	Total
Alcohol	70	91	161
Drugs	5	156	161

TABLE 9.22
Type of Social Setting

Setting	Number
Informal	151
Formal	10
Total	161

governmental agencies or find it difficult to do so. There were seven (4.3%) additional ocean diving injuries, but they occurred off of piers, docks, and jetties.

SUBSTANCE ABUSE

Table 9.21 describes related substance abuse. Victims acknowledged they had consumed some form of alcoholic beverage (mostly beer) sometime during the day of the accident in 70(43.5%) of the cases. Only five (3.1%) victims admitted to being under the influence of drugs.

TYPE OF SOCIAL SETTING

The social setting in which the accident occurred is summarized in Table 9.22. The gathering was informal in 151 (93.8%) cases. On only ten (6.2%) occasions was the event planned in advance with written or verbal invitations. These were most often company parties.

TABLE 9.23
Posted Rules and Warning Signs

Instructions	Yes	No	Total
Posted rules	56	105	161
Warning signs	12	149	161

TABLE 9.24
Lifeguard on Duty

Lifeguard	Number
Yes	29
No	132
Total	161

TABLE 9.25
Person Making Rescue

Rescuer	Number
Friends	140
Lifeguard	12
EMS	7
Self	2
Total	161

TABLE 9.26
Use of Spineboard and CPR

Technique	Yes	No	Total
Spineboard	10	151	161
CPR	30	131	161

TABLE 9.27
Paramedics Involved

Technique	Number
Yes	136
No	25
Total	161

SAFETY AND SUPERVISION

POSTED RULES AND WARNING SIGNS

Table 9.23 indicates the extent to which rules for the use of the facility were posted and the number of sites that contained warning signs against diving. Even though nearly half of the 161 accident sites were designated for swimming (see Table 9.9), 105(65.2%) had no rules posted instructing users concerning their conduct. Only 12(7.5%) of the accident sites had any warning signs prohibiting diving.

LIFEGUARD ON DUTY

A lifeguard was on duty at 29(18.0%) of the accident locations, as shown in Table 9.24.

RESCUE PROCEDURES

The final four tables again indicate the need for educating people as to the proper procedures to follow when a person is suspected of having a spinal cord injury.

PERSON MAKING RESCUE

The person making the rescue is presented in Table 9.25. Friends of the victim or other swimmers who were nearby made 140(87.0%) of the rescues. Lifeguards performed 12(7.5%), emergency medical services (EMS) performed 7(4.3%), and victims were responsible for 2(1.2%) rescues.

USE OF SPINEBOARD AND CARDIOPULMONARY RESUSCITATION

The most disturbing fact revealed in Table 9.26 shows that in only ten (6.2%) cases was the victim removed from the water by use of a spineboard. This means that the vast majority were lifted, pulled, or dragged out of the water by friends who were not aware of the injury to the spinal cord. Cardiopulmonary resuscitation (CPR) was used in only 30(18.6%) of the cases. This indicates that most victims were rescued within the first two minutes, and were still breathing.

PARAMEDIC INVOLVEMENT

Paramedics were involved in 136(84.5%) of the accidents, as shown in Table 9.27. When compared with Table 9.26, however, it is clear that the vast majority of the time they arrived after the initial rescue was accomplished.

SUMMARY OF FACTS

The following facts were derived from the data presented in this chapter.

- The young adult male is at greatest risk.
- The victim had no formal diving instruction during his lifetime.
- Some form of alcoholic beverage had been consumed in 70 (43.4%) cases.
- Of the 161 cases, 5(3.1%) victims may have been under the influence of drugs.
- Invariably the person was injured on his first visit to the accident site.
- In 130(80.7%) of the cases, the victim was injured on his first dive.
- Compression fracture in the C-5 and C-6 area was the most prevalent injury level.
- None of the victims received a fracture of the skull.
- Most victims did not require rescue breathing or CPR.
- Almost all victims were rescued by friends or other swimmers who did not use a spineboard.
- The depth of water where the victim struck the bottom was less than 4 ft.
- There were no signs warning against diving in the area where the dive occurred.
- There were no rules posted restricting use of the area.
- A dock or pier extending out into a lake or ocean was the primary location of dives resulting in the injury. Most occurred either at the end of the dock or pier or off the side (Figures 9.1 and 9.2).
- No lifeguard was on duty in the area where the dive was made.
- Almost all the accidents occurred in a designated swimming area.

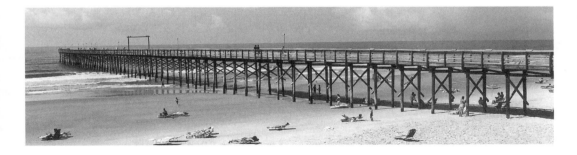

FIGURE 9.1 Piers and docks extending into oceans present an invitation to dive or jump.

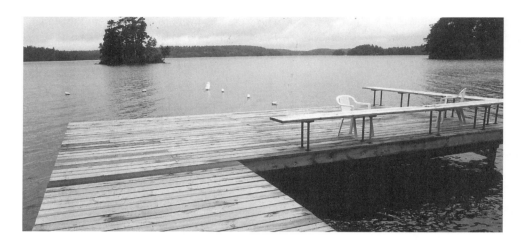

FIGURE 9.2 More diving injuries occur from people diving off private docks located on lakes.

CONCLUSIONS

Many of the diving injuries, in our opinion, could have been prevented if owners of the areas and aquatic facilities had followed known principles of aquatic safety. Far too much emphasis is placed on the responsibility of the diver. It is necessary to look critically at how these water areas and facilities are managed and operated. The following factors stand out from the analysis of the 161 diving injuries that occurred in the natural environment.

MAJOR FACTORS CONTRIBUTING TO DIVING ACCIDENTS

A careful examination of where these accidents occurred and the circumstances surrounding them led us to conclude that the factors listed next were major contributors to the accidents.

Shallow Water

Shallow water was the major cause of the injuries. The depth where the dive was made was too shallow (under 4 ft) to safely permit diving.

Turbid Water Conditions

The water was so turbid (muddy and cloudy) that the bottom was not visible. Objects such as rocks, dead trees, and ledges lying on the bottom could not be seen.

Inexperienced Diver

Most of the victims had received no formal training in diving and had participated in diving from only a recreational point of view. They were not aware of the dangers associated with diving into unknown waters and were motivated to dive by the urging of friends and by seeing others dive before them.

Diver Misjudgment

The diver's misjudgment of the conditions that existed in the area of the intended dive were, in most instances, the depth of water and overestimating his ability to execute a safe dive.

Failure of Property Owners

Owners with water on or adjacent to their land had failed to post warning signs citing the dangers and hazards that existed and prohibiting diving in certain areas to those entering their property.

Unsupervised Recreation Areas

Owners of hotels or city/state parks often permit people to boat, swim, and dive in lakes and rivers adjacent to, or on, their property without providing any instruction to, or supervision of, users.

Failure to Inform and Warn

Owners and operators of aquatic areas and facilities failed to post signs prohibiting diving in certain areas and to adequately inform, instruct, and warn users of the potential dangers that existed. (See Chapter 13.)

Lack of Lifeguards in Designated Swimming Areas

Contrary to the belief of many people, most of the diving accidents occurred in designated swimming areas. However, in only 29(18.0%) situations were lifeguards on duty at the time of the accident.

Lack of Risk Analysis

The practice of commercial enterprises (resort hotels and beaches) not having a risk analysis made to identify existing hazards before offering their facilities to patrons and permitting swimming is inexcusable.

Failure to Remove Trees and Branches

Owners of water property—both public and private—are irresponsible when they fail to remove branches of trees or trees themselves to which youths have attached ropes for swinging into the water. (Figure 9.3).

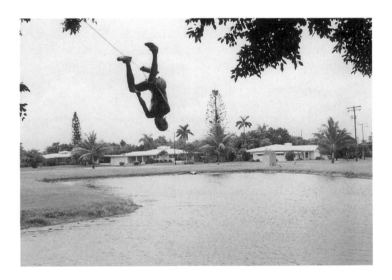

FIGURE 9.3 Four youths were injured swinging off ropes attached to trees.

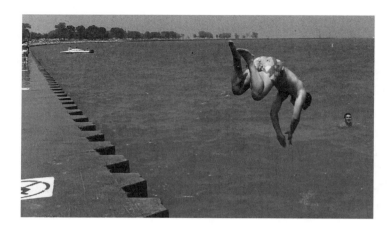

FIGURE 9.4 Diving off walls can be dangerous.

Misplaced Structures

The placement of structures into, adjacent to, or over water areas can create a potentially dangerous condition. Owners and operators must recognize and take the steps to prevent accidents from occurring on or off structures such as docks extending into lakes, rivers, or the ocean; bridges or bulkheads at water's edge; and rafts (Figure 9.4).

Lack of Public Education

If diving accidents are to be reduced, the population must be educated about the dangers of diving into unfamiliar waters and instructed as to the precautions that must be taken before entering the water. Such admonitions as "Look before you leap" and "Feet first the first time" have had positive effects on people.

Running Dives from Beaches

Diving into the ocean by running from the beach and launching oneself headfirst into a wave can be dangerous if the dive is too shallow and the wave breaks down on the diver. When diving into the ocean one should dive through an incoming wave, not under it (Figure 9.5).

MOST DANGEROUS ACTIVITIES

The most dangerous types of activities made into water areas other than swimming pools are:

- Diving from cliffs or high embankments adjacent to the shore of rivers and lakes (Figure 9.6)
- Diving from bridges
- Diving from high piers located on oceanfronts
- Diving from boat docks that extend out into a lake or river
- Diving from a retaining wall or bulkhead
- Diving from boats into water that is too shallow
- Swinging from a rope attached to a branch of a tree extending over the water

DEFICIENCIES NOTED IN THE DESIGN, OPERATION, AND USE OF AQUATIC FACILITIES

A critical examination of the findings recorded in this chapter, visits to the accident scenes, and discussions with many of the victims have provided the authors with an insight into some of the

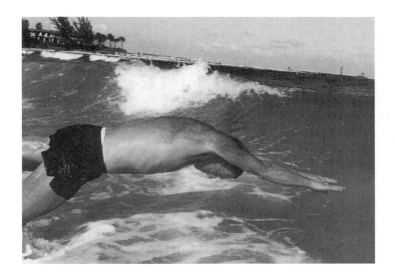

FIGURE 9.5 Running dive into ocean waves.

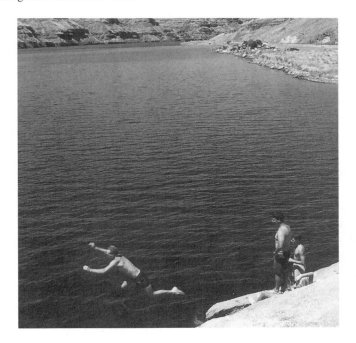

FIGURE 9.6 Jumping or diving off cliffs is exceedingly dangerous.

causative factors related to the diving injuries occurring in our lakes, rivers, oceans, and other water areas. The following conclusions were derived from analyses of the data presented in this chapter.

Failure of Owners and Operators to Follow Known Principles of Aquatic Safety

Failure of owners and operators of parks, resort hotels, campgrounds, public beaches, motels, commercial beaches, and vacation homes to follow basic principles of aquatic safety in the planning, design, and operation of aquatic facilities includes the following:

1. To survey or have surveyed the water and surrounding area supporting the beach facility to determine:

   - Toxicity of water
   - Bacterial content of water
   - Composition of bottom of proposed swimming area
   - Slope of bottom
   - Water condition (muddy, presence of algae, marine life)
   - Presence of currents (annual/seasonal)
   - Fluctuations of water level
   - Underwater obstructions
   - Presence of drop-offs and holes
   - Safe swimming and diving areas

2. To prepare plans (architectural or engineering) of the swimming beach that would establish:

   - Safe swimming area
   - Area for nonswimmers and children
   - Safest area for boating, if boating is to be allowed
   - Location of a water skiing area and other power-operated equipment
   - Specifications for installation of docks for boating, swimming, and diving indicating their design, height, and location
   - Recommended signage necessary to inform patrons of water depths, safe use of areas, and dangers that may be present and need to be guarded against

3. To establish policies and procedures outlined next for the management, operation, and maintenance of the aquatic facilities under their control and the people who use them:

   - Posting rules for the use of the beach at all entrances to the beach
   - Posting separate rules for boating, water skiing, fishing, and other activities conducted away from the swimming beach
   - Hiring certified lifeguards and assigning them to supervise patrons and to enforce beach rules and regulations
   - Placing lifeguards in stands with telephone or radio communication
   - Ensuring that there is proper lifesaving and rescue equipment present on the beach
   - Prohibiting people from swimming at the beach when lifeguards are not on duty— especially important at night to have night security lights on the beach to help detect intruders
   - Establishing means for enforcing rules
   - Posting warning signs at locations where diving is prohibited
   - Ensuring at all times (night or day) that there will be someone on the staff trained and qualified to administer first aid and CPR if necessary

Failure of Patrons to Act Safely in the Use of Designated Swimming Facilities

The following represent some of the actions of patrons (users) that have led to injury:

1. Disregarding/disobeying

   - Warning signs
   - Posted rules
   - Lifeguard instructions

2. Failing to

 • Determine water depth in the area where a dive is contemplated
 • Make entry feet first at the time of initial entry into any water that is unfamiliar to the diver
 • Have head and arms in proper alignment with the body
 • Accurately determine the depth of water where the dive is contemplated

3. Lack of training and awareness of diver to

 • Recognize the effect that running and diving from platforms or docks higher than 12 in. above the water have on entry velocity (see Figures 9.1 and 9.2).
 • Understand the mechanics of diving
 • Understand the danger relative to diving into shallow water
 • Know what water depth is safe for diving

4. Other

 • Following the actions of another person
 • Running down a beach or shore into the water and launching into a dive where the water is too shallow (see Figure 9.5).
 • Diving while under the influence of alcohol or drugs
 • Going down a high slide headfirst (see Figure 9.7)
 • Overestimating the ability to dive from unfamiliar locations

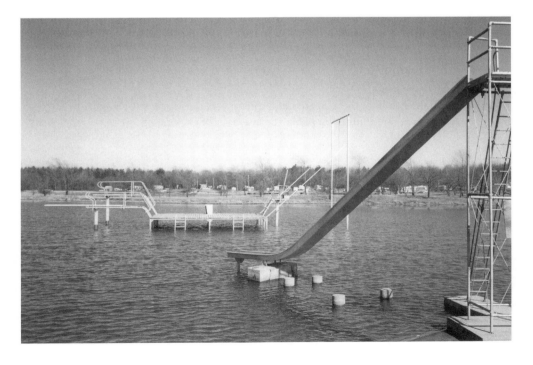

FIGURE 9.7 High slides into shallow water have resulted in serious injuries.

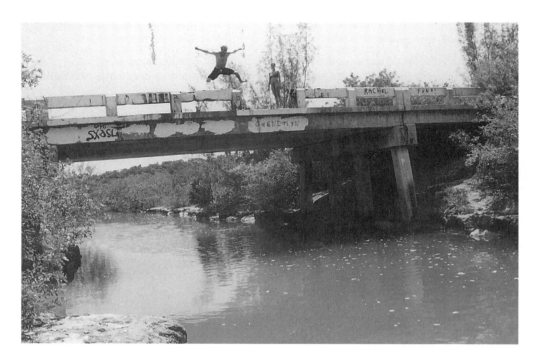

FIGURE 9.8 Diving off bridges caused several injuries.

Failure of Commercial Builders and/or Contractors

Commercial builders and/or contractors may fail in the following ways:

1. To warn people against swimming and diving in their excavations (by posting signs)
2. To fence

   • Construction areas
   • Canals or ponds that they created and that are located adjacent to apartment/condominium complexes or a housing development

3. To remove

   • Equipment that is close to the edge of, or in, the water
   • Trees and overhanging branches located at shoreline to prevent youngsters from hanging a rope for swinging (see Figure 9.3)

4. To recognize teenagers and young adults as being attracted to newly created water areas

Failure to Educate the Public in the Selection of Safe Swimming Areas

Without a doubt, more people are injured by diving into water that is not designated as an official swimming area including:

   • Bridges
   • Canals

- Cliffs
- Farm ponds
- Lakes in parks
- Quarries
- Reservoirs
- Shorelines of inland lakes and rivers
- Unguarded ocean beaches

People get to these water areas usually by walking or driving. Others arrive by canoes, various types of boats, rubber rafts, planes, and other modes of transportation. They are on their own once they get to the facility with only their prior training, experience, and knowledge to guide them in their selection of, and participation in, certain water activities. The transfer of ability acquired in one setting to another is not always automatic. For example, having acquired the skill to dive from a 1-m-high springboard does not guarantee that the diver will be able to execute a safe dive from a 10-ft-high cliff bordering a river or lake.

Regulation of how people should use these water areas or what owners should be required to do is most often impractical and unrealistic. One essential way to have any effect on how people use these undeveloped and undesignated swimming areas is to educate them in the proper use of these areas, particularly with respect to identifying the activities that are dangerous. Some of the activities that people commonly participate in that can lead to an injury are

1. Diving into shallow water (less than 5 ft) from

   - Bridges
   - Seawall or bulkhead
   - Embankments next to rivers or lakes
   - Cliffs 10 to 20 ft high
   - Branches of overhanging trees
   - Boats
   - Boat docks and piers (Figure 9.9)

2. Swinging on ropes attached to trees
3. Running on the ground to the edge of a bank and diving into the ocean or waves

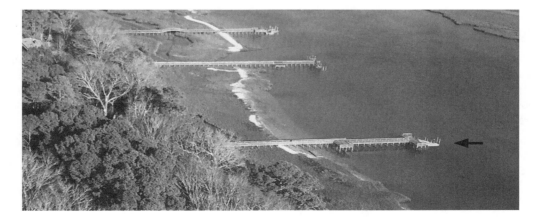

FIGURE 9.9 Long docks give a false impression of water depth.

Failure of Owners of Vacation Homes and Cottages

Whenever a boat dock is constructed it should be anticipated that young people might attempt to dive from it. Where the water is less than 5 ft deep, diving should be prohibited and guests should be informed both verbally and by appropriate signs placed at the beginning (approach) to the dock, along the edge of the sides of the dock, and at the end of the dock. (See Chapter 13.)

Failure of Sponsors and Organizers of Groups that Use Aquatic Areas

All parks at every level—city/county and state/federal facilities, and private campgrounds—have organized groups who visit and use these sites. This may be a one-day or picnic-type activity or it may be a camping activity where the group stays for a week or more. Examples of groups include schools, colleges, Girl and Boy Scouts, Boys' Clubs, Ys, employers, and religious organizations.

One of the essential steps for every organization taking youngsters or adults to aquatic areas is the need to plan properly for the total program. Planning starts long before the event. Preplanning involves establishing the program and assessing the need for any specialized, experienced leadership to conduct the activities. Of all the activities that are usually involved in a program, those related to water such as swimming, diving, scuba diving, and boating are some of the more dangerous and need careful planning to ensure the safety of the participants.

Frequent errors in this process include the failure to

1. **Plan,** in advance, the selection of an appropriate site to accommodate the activities that will be made available to those attending the outing
2. **Visit,** in advance, the site where the group will be going on the outing
3. **Assess** the dangers and risks that exist in and around the area, and adjust planned activities as necessary
4. **Act** by taking the steps necessary to ensure the safety of the participants, which may include the prohibition of activities that are potentially dangerous and the provision of additional staff necessary to supervise participants

RECOMMMENDATIONS

Based on the data presented in this chapter and the conclusions we have reached, the following recommendations are made in an attempt to reduce the number of these catastrophic injuries.

PUBLIC EDUCATION

Greater effort must be made to educate the public with respect to water safety so that people intending to swim in water bodies located in the natural environment will know what steps must be taken to prevent injury from diving and drowning of any member of the group. Every means possible should be used to reach the public with information that will enable it to enjoy our water areas and facilities without injury. Some of the means that should be used are:

- Television spots on water safety
- Radio programs on the subject of water safety
- News releases on water safety prepared by agencies such as the ARC, Council for National Cooperation in Aquatics, Consumer Product Safety Commission (CPSC), national parks, Coast Guard, and others that have a role to play

- Preparation and dissemination of videocassettes for home use on various aspects of water safety
- A 30-minute segment on water safety should be included in the curriculum at every grade in school throughout the 12 years, and instructional material should be prepared by schools to meet local needs with the assistance of professional groups

RESPONSIBLE DESIGN, OWNERSHIP, AND OPERATION

All those who own, construct, develop, and offer aquatic facilities to the public must assume the responsibility for making them as safe as possible. This includes the proper design of aquatic areas and facilities, the supervision of users by qualified personnel, and the operation of areas to ensure the safety of participants. To achieve this safety, the following must be accomplished:

- Educating and instructing the public by every means possible
- Communicating with users through warning and instructional signs
- Inspecting all aquatic areas and facilities on a regular basis
- Providing qualified lifeguards and supervisors for the safety of patrons

PROFESSIONAL STANDARDS

Professional groups and agencies that manage aquatic facilities need to develop standards for their layout, design, and operation.

BOAT DOCK STANDARDS

Some types of standards, or at least guidelines, need to be developed to regulate the design, installation, and operation of boat docks. Factors, such as the height and width of the dock, need for depth markers, and signs prohibiting diving where the water is not deep enough to safely accommodate diving, need to be addressed because it is apparent that many of the injuries occurring each year are the result of people diving from docks extending out into lakes and rivers (see Figures 9.1 and 9.2).

A PLEA FROM VICTIMS

One of the opportunities available to the authors was the chance to meet and interview many of the accident victims. It was disturbing to hear them say that they had no idea that they could break their neck where they made their dive. They were also very adamant that if someone had told them or there had been a sign posted prohibiting diving, they would not have made the dive.

Finally, they pointed out that they believed the site to be safe for diving because of certain features giving the appearance of deep water and their observation of other divers. All this adds up to the need to make every effort to communicate with the general public to increase awareness of the hazards and potential dangers that exist in the natural water environment.

10 Mathematics and Mechanics of Diving

INTRODUCTION

This chapter examines the mechanics and mathematics of diving, and the causes of these injuries from springboards and low takeoffs (such as those from pool decks and docks). Readers are urged to review Chapters 5 to 8 to learn how these diving injuries occurred. In addition, Appendix B contains illustrations of some of the research that was conducted at Nova Southeastern University's Dive/Slide Research Center.

To be able to properly assess what affects a diver's performance, it is essential to understand the mechanics of diving and the various factors that may affect performance. This discussion is divided into these three parts:

- Diving from springboards and platforms
- Diving from low-fixed platforms such as from the deck of a pool, a starting block used in swimming competition, or a structure such as a dock
- Headfirst slides on water slides

In some areas comments have been made on the variations in performance between the trained and untrained person to illustrate why or how the untrained diver may be inadvertently placed in a dangerous posture (i.e., in the execution of a shallow-type dive into water too shallow for safety).

SPRINGBOARD AND PLATFORM DIVING

The diver's performance from springboards or high, stationary platforms is influenced by external conditions or certain human factors. Each factor mentioned may adversely affect the performance.

EXTERNAL FACTORS

Type of Springboard

The length, width, design, construction, and resultant spring or flexibility of the board are all significant factors. Aluminum boards, being the most flexible, provide the highest performance and are used primarily in competitive diving today. Wooden and fiberglass boards are less flexible; nevertheless, they provide considerable thrust and spring, particularly when adults use them. The board stores and returns additional energy that helps project the diver up and forward, away from the end of the board.

Condition of the Board

This includes slipperiness of its surface, torque in the board, cracks, deterioration of its original properties, and absence or presence of a protective covering at the end of the board.

Installation of the Board

Important factors include anchors, fittings, levelness, position of the fulcrum, alignment, distance the board extends over the edge of the pool, distance between the board and adjacent springboards, protective guard rails on the side of the stand, height of the board from the water, and distance from any overhead obstructions.

Board Response

This includes the quickness of the board in response to the diver's depression of the board, which may range from the soft deep movement of the modern aluminum board to the fast, hard, and short flexion of the shorter wood and fiberglass boards. Board response is also related to the position of the fulcrum. The farther back the fulcrum is positioned, the deeper the board flexion will be, although it will be slower in response.

Environmental Conditions

Both springboard and platform divers may be adversely affected by environmental factors, including glare from the sun or from outside light in the case of indoor pools, pool width, depth of the water in the diving area, bottom contours, presence of bottom markings, intensity of illumination, wind velocities, location of light sources, and turbidity of the water. Platforms for diving are usually 20 ft in length and extend $2\frac{1}{2}$ ft or more over the water depending on height. Normal platform heights are 3, 5, 7.5, or 10 m above the water surface. An adequate volume of water is essential to safely accommodate dives from any height. Untrained or recreational divers need more water volume than do trained or competitive divers. Untrained or recreational divers tend to dive out and away from the takeoff point compared with trained or competitive divers who tend to dive up and close (Figure 10.1). Obviously, untrained divers make more errors when diving and display considerably more inconsistency in the process.

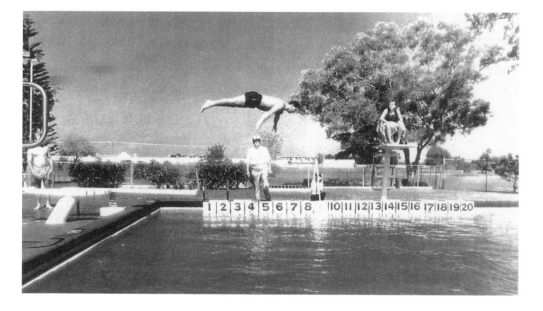

FIGURE 10.1 A recreational diver going way out because of the angle when leaving the board.

HUMAN FACTORS

Physiological Characteristics and Condition of the Diver

These include weight, height, center of gravity, body proportions, strength, visual acuity, fatigue, drug or alcohol consumption, and any weakness that may have been caused by illness or physical disabilities.

Ability and Agility of the Diver

The experience, training, neuromuscular coordination, and general athletic ability of the diver affects performance.

Psychological Factors

Personal fear, hesitation, peer pressure, tendency to show off, "freezing up," mental lapses, unfamiliar circumstances, disorientation caused by distractions or noise originating from around the pool, personality dynamics, and emotional stability of the diver are factors that could be adverse elements affecting safety as well as performance.

COMPONENTS INVOLVED IN EXECUTING A DIVE

STARTING POSITION

Assumed by the diver prior to beginning the dive, the starting position may be at the end of the board or platform facing out toward the water (standing dives) or facing inward from the end of the board (backward and inward dives). Most forward dives performed on springboards and platforms, however, are begun with a forward moving approach from the back of the springboard or platform toward the front end.

APPROACH

The diver walks slowly toward the front end of the board, placing himself in a position for the "hurdle." In the platform approach, a run is generally used. Some authorities refer to the approach as the "steps." Most trained divers, when using a 16-ft competitive board, use the three- or four-step "walking" approach before making the hurdle. The inexperienced diver is more apt to run.

HURDLE AND BOARD DEPRESSION

The most crucial step in the execution of a good dive, the hurdle, brings the diver's body to a height above the board (see Figure 14.6). The diver then drops onto the end of the board with the weight of the body, causing the board to be depressed and to store energy. The heavier the body is, the greater the depression will be. The extent to which the board is depressed is determined by five factors: (1) the height the diver achieves above the board during the hurdle, (2) the body weight, (3) the leg flexion, (4) the strength of the legs, and (5) the flexibility of the board (see Figure 14.7). The hurdle and board depression can be compared with that of a slingshot, which when drawn back stores the energy necessary to send out a projectile. Coupling a board with the diver's hurdle and takeoff thrust essentially causes a doubling of the energy associated with the dive. The stored energy in the depressed board acts with the momentum transfer (i.e., leg and arm thrust) of the diver to provide increased time during flight. This is a result of the height reached, after takeoff, by the diver's center of mass, which is located in the vicinity of the hips and waist.

TAKEOFF

This phase of the dive determines the vertical, horizontal, and lateral direction the diver takes. As the diver lands on the end of the board from the hurdle, the knees are bent as the board is depressed to obtain maximum effectiveness. As the board is being depressed, the diver brings the arms down to the sides of the body. The diver is now in a coiled or crouched position, following which the proper application of arm lift, added to the energy supplied by the board flexion and extension of the diver's legs, projects the body up and away from the board in a parabolic arc. This specific combination and coordination of movements separate the skilled diver from the novice. These movements are embedded in the skilled diver's learning so that concentration can be centered on the planned execution during the flight in air (see Figure 14.8).

All diving is a form of somersaulting. In the proper takeoff, the body alignment of the diver is forward from the vertical. This angle is essential to avoid striking the board, for if the diver is "dead vertical" he will go straight up and return to the same spot of the takeoff. Furthermore, it is the forward lean at takeoff that provides the essential rotation or angular momentum of the body necessary for the execution of dives.

The untrained diver, unfamiliar with the mechanics of the hurdle and liftoff, invariably approaches to the end of the board with a longer hurdle and with greater speed than are necessary or desirable. These factors provide a forward momentum that often causes the novice to lean forward excessively on the liftoff. When an untrained diver combines a forward lean with a good board depression, strong and effective leg action, and good arm lift, the dive can result in achieving considerable distance horizontally from the end of the board (Figure 10.2). This reaction is likely to place the diver in a dangerous location at water entry, particularly if a safe water depth does not extend forward of the board sufficiently enough to provide a safe landing and maneuvering area.

Diving research conducted at Nova University has demonstrated that an adult person with average athletic skill, using a springboard that is 24 in. above the water and only 12 ft long, can be projected a distance of 14 to 16 ft from the end of the board before entering the water (Figure 10.3). In a spoon-shaped or hopper-bottom-type pool, the diver almost always enters the water where the depth is considerably less than that existing at the deepest point.

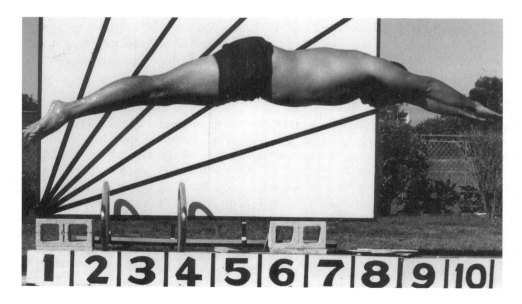

FIGURE 10.2 A 220-lb 6 ft 2 in. recreational diver being projected out from the board.

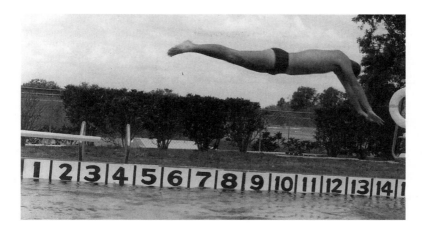

FIGURE 10.3 Diver going up and out from a 12-ft-long springboard, 24 in. above the water.

FLIGHT OF THE BODY

A diver's center of mass follows a special in-air trajectory after liftoff from the board. Nothing the diver does while in flight can change that trajectory. The center of mass travels in a parabolic arc, decelerating on the way up, until the body literally stops in its vertical motion at the top of the arc (see Figure 10.2). The energy that produces the diver's velocity on the downward flight is derived from the earth's gravitational attraction. The diver reaches a near maximum velocity at the point of entry into the water.

During the flight through the air, the diver may execute a variety of motions called "dives." These motions range from the simple dives of the untrained person to complex somersaults, twists, and reverses (or a combination of these) performed by the trained diver. For example, a diver may perform a one and one half forward somersault with a double twist. Accomplishing these movement variations requires great body control, which can be achieved only with practice, concentration, and fine muscular coordination. The good diver never closes his eyes until entering the water.

BODY ENTRY

Most diving instructors recommend an entry into the water that is short of vertical. The entry may be head first with arms extended overhead protecting the head, or it may be feet first with arms placed at the sides of the body. The less than vertical entry tends to compensate for the tendency of the body to continue its rotation after the head enters the water. Divers have often been observed going "over" on a dive. That is, angular momentum kept the legs moving forward so that they "flopped" over. For the inexperienced diver, that is a common error. Conversely, if the angle of entry is too "short," the diver might well land on the stomach (see Figure 14.9).

COURSE OF THE BODY IN WATER

In the perfect entry and subsequent transition through the water, the trained diver holds the entry position until the hands strike the bottom, or in a deep pool, until the velocity decreases sufficiently to enable a maneuver to return to the surface. An entry of this type is labeled a "clean" entry. There is little, if any, break in the body alignment until the diver is immersed in the water.

An experienced diver often alters the in-water trajectory to correct a "going over" or short in-air trajectory. Such maneuvers are commonly referred to as a "save." These movements involve a quick arching of the back and raising of the head for back and reverse spinning dives, or rotating in water in a continuing somersault for forward and inward dives.

When the body is in alignment, or nearly so, with the trajectory of the center of mass with the arms properly extended above the head, no deceleration occurs during the first 2 to 3 ft of water entry. In fact, the speed of the diver's head increases for a short time after penetration of the water. Studies of high-speed motion picture photography have shown that the speed of the diver's head is essentially the same as at the surface of the water when about three fourths of the body is immersed (see Figure 14.10).

DIVING FROM LOW STATIONARY STRUCTURES

More people are injured when diving from low heights such as the deck of a pool, appurtenances and objects placed near pools, starting blocks, and docks and piers that extend into lakes and rivers than are injured from springboards. The ratio is about 5:1 according to the data reported in Chapter 4. However, the number of dives performed from the deck of a pool or other low structures as compared with springboards is much greater. There is, however, a general under-estimation by the recreational diver of the hazard and risk involved in diving from low heights into water too shallow for safety. Because of prior experience, recreational swimmers/divers tend to overestimate their abilities and underestimate the danger. See Figures 10.4 and 10.5 illustrating safe body alignment above and below the water when performing shallow dives from the deck of a pool.

The elements involved in executing a dive from the pool deck or any stationary low-fixed object described earlier are basically the same as those involved in a springboard dive. The principle exception is the energy source. In springboard diving an additional energy source is provided by the board, while in diving from a stationary position the energy is generated solely by the diver. Most of the kinetic energy comes from the thrust of the legs. However, when used properly, the arms can add significantly to the energy. Once the diver is in the air, gravitational attraction takes over, bringing the diver down to the water. The various components involved in performing a headfirst standing dive from the side of a pool or from a dock may be characterized as follows:

- Initial static position the diver assumes at the start of the dive
- Leg flexion and thrust at takeoff
- Lifting power generated by the arms
- Flight trajectory of the diver's body as it passes through the air
- Angle of the diver's body as it enters the water

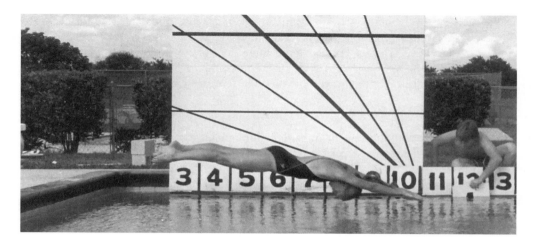

FIGURE 10.4 Illustrates a flat, shallow dive.

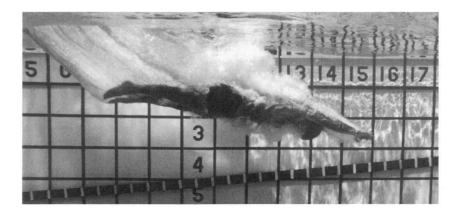

FIGURE 10.5 Correct underwater body alignment for a shallow dive.

- In-water path the diver takes and body alignment
- Position of the arms and head during the diver's in-water path

The position of the head at water entry is of particular concern when considering diving into water too shallow. Inexperienced divers drop their heads at entry into the water to take the impact of water entry on the top of the head instead of on the face. However, if the head is not lifted after water entry and the back is not arched, this head position can cause a downward rotation. Thus, if a diver delays lifting the head and arching the back, the in-water trajectory is deeper than planned. In shallow water environments, impact with the bottom at traumatic injury–producing speeds can be the result. This effect is due to Newton's third law of motion (i.e., the action–reaction law) and can best be experienced by "flying" one's hand outside of a moving automobile. A slight lifting or lowering of the hand causes the hand and arm to suddenly be moved to a trailing position in the wind stream. Because of the wide variations in performance among recreational swimmers/divers, diving into water too shallow must be prohibited.

A running dive from the edge of a pool or dock (as opposed to a dive from a standing start) involves all the preceding components with the exception of the initial static position, which becomes a dynamic position. The speed of the run combined with the vigor of the takeoff can result in the diver being projected farther out from the edge of the pool or dock and traveling at a higher velocity than that achieved when performing a standing dive.

The crucial factor associated with diving into shallow water is the element of time. From research studies conducted at Nova University, it has been established that a person diving from a low height and entering the water at an angle of 45 degrees in a pool 3.5 ft deep strikes the bottom in less than a half second after the head touches the surface of the water. If the hands and arms are not "locked" and in a correct position to deflect and/or absorb the impact of striking the bottom, the diver may be seriously injured. Because the time interval is so short (i.e., less than that needed for reaction/response time for a "surprise" event), proper "programming" of the diver's trajectory must take place prior to executing the dive. In other words, the diver must program the lifting of the head and the arching of the back immediately after entry into water too shallow.

SLIDING HEADFIRST DOWN A WATER SLIDE

Sliding headfirst down a water-lubricated slide is similar to diving except for the fact that the energy producer is the height of the slide instead of the springboard, and the slide bed restricts the range of body movements. The higher the slide is, the greater the gravitational energy potential and the resultant velocity of the body at water entry. It has been demonstrated by photographic analysis conducted at Nova University that slides as low as 4 to 6 ft provide sufficient velocities to precipitate a serious injury-producing event should impact occur in shallow water.

The principal elements related to the position and characteristics of the slide are the overall height of the slide, the vertical height of the exit ramp above the water's surface, the angle and curvature of the slide bed, and the friction of the slide bed surface. The two most significant injury-contributing factors are (1) the depth of water immediately under the slide exit and out to a horizontal distance of 16 ft in front of the slide, and (2) what the slider does after exit from the slide and during the in-water travel. The slider should be prepared to enter the water with palms and head in an "up" position with the back slightly arched. The slider must not drop the head or "break" at the waist when exiting from the slide. In feet-first entries following a descent in a sitting position, the legs must not be dropped or they may strike the bottom. Because of the danger associated with headfirst slides and their similarity to diving, water slides should not be installed where one would not install a diving board.

Height of Slide Exit Ramp Above Water

The higher the exit ramp of the slide is above the water, the more the slider can alter body alignment and body component configuration, thereby inducing an in-water downward rotation. The higher the exit ramp is above the water, the greater the increase in the vertical velocity of the slider.

Exit Angle of Slide

The nearer the exit angle is to horizontal and the closer the exit ramp is to the water, the more likely it is that the slider can make a safe, shallow entry into the water. The Nova University study indicated that the longer the exit portion of the slide, the more likely the body of the slider will be placed at a proper angle for water entry.

Angle of Water Entry

Any water entry into shallow water where the upper trunk is inclined downward toward the water can result in contact with the bottom at injury-producing speeds. To avoid such impact, the slider must take immediate action before and during entry into water to change the in-water path to a more shallow trajectory. This is achieved by raising the head and arching the back. As stated previously, these actions must be "programmed" by the slider prior to initiating the slide because of the very short time between water entry and potential impact with the bottom.

In-Water Speeds

The in-water velocity a slider achieves is primarily determined by the speed and angle of entry established by the starting height, friction, design of the slide, and hydrodynamic drag of the body. The slider achieves a maximum in-water speed if body alignment is held in a clean entry position. The head speed achieved at a 3-ft depth when sliders in the Nova University studies entered at a near vertical angle from slides 6 to 12 ft high ranged from 14.5 to 27 ft/s.

Hydrodynamic Drag

Every slider's in-water speed is affected by hydrodynamic drag. This drag force is primarily determined by cross-sectional body area and speed squared. After water entry, hydrodynamic drag is the only force that acts to slow a slider executing a clean trajectory.

Depth of Penetration

How deep a person goes as a result of going down a water slide in a headfirst position is determined by body angle at water entry, body alignment, speed at water entry, and hydrodynamic drag.

Studies have revealed that sliders of adult size who held straight body alignment had little difficulty going down to the bottom in a pool 12 ft deep. In a deeper pool, some sliders had sufficient momentum to carry them down to a depth of 18 ft after descending an 8-foot-high slide in a headfirst position.

MECHANICAL CONSIDERATIONS

CENTER OF MASS

An understanding of the physical laws associated with body motion permits us to use the concept of "center of mass." During translational motion, each point on the body undergoes the same displacement as another. Thus, the motion of one point, the center of the mass, is representative of the entire body's motion. Even if the body should rotate or twist, its center of mass always moves in the same way that a single particle would move if it were subjected to the identical external forces, such as gravitational attraction. In a typical human body, the center of mass is located in the vicinity of the hips and waist.

AIR RESISTANCE AND WIND

Air resistance is negligible for dives or water-lubricated slides from heights up to 10 m above the water. Unless the wind is blowing quite strongly, it does not affect divers using boards and platforms placed at normal heights (i.e., up to 10 m) because of the short free fall time. However, the wind may have a psychological effect on divers.

ENERGY SOURCE

A diver executing a standing dive from a stationary object derives energy from two sources: leg and arm thrust plus gravitational attraction. Much is known relative to the ability of high school and college-age students to jump vertically off the ground. In experimental studies, Gerrish,[1] Considine and Sullivan,[2] and Offenbacher[3] found that the height reached by the center of mass of the average college student in a free-standing jump averaged about 21 in. with a standard deviation of 3 in. Batterman[4] found that an expert diver, using a hurdle jump, could raise his center of mass to about 30 in. Thus, it can be reasonably assumed that an untrained, adult-sized diver is quite capable of executing a standing vertical jump to heights ranging from 12 to 24 in. This is equivalent to an initial velocity at takeoff ranging from 8.0 to 11.3 ft/s. (5.4 to 7.7 m/h). Unless a diver literally falls off the platform, there is both a horizontal and vertical (upward) movement of the center of mass. The result is a parabolic trajectory of the center of mass while in free fall. The more athletic a person is, the higher and longer the trajectory through the air is likely to be.

DIRECTION AND TRAJECTORY IN AIR

Once the diver leaves the springboard or platform, the direction and trajectory of the dive are fixed in the air. The trajectory has the form of a parabola, $y = ax - bx^2$. Nothing the diver does while undergoing flight can result in a change in the direction or the trajectory of the center of mass.

MAXIMUM HEIGHT OF DIVER'S TRAJECTORY ABOVE WATER

A trained diver, using a high-performance 16-ft aluminum springboard, can achieve a height of as much as 8 ft above the board. When using a 10- to 12-ft-long fiberglass board, heights of 6 to 7 ft above the board can be attained. A Nova University photographic study of an untrained diver, weighing 200 lb and 6 ft 2 in. (74 in.) in height revealed that the subject could easily raise his center of mass to heights of 6 to 8 ft above a fiberglass springboard that was 10 ft long.

Leg and arm thrusts provide energy additional to that returned by the springboard. The height of the center of mass above the water at the highest point in the diver's trajectory involves the height of the springboard or platform above the water, the energy derived from the spring of the board, and the diver's jumping ability and takeoff angle.

WATER ENTRY POINT

The distance from the end of a springboard or platform to the water entry point is determined by (1) physical characteristics/capabilities of the diver; (2) diver's takeoff angle, direction, and takeoff speed; (3) flexibility of the board; and (4) height of the springboard or platform above the water. Increasing the horizontal velocity component and the flight time in the air results in greater distances from the board. Although off-axis dives from a springboard or platform may not achieve the same distances as on-axis dives, the resultant trajectories in water may nevertheless result in contact with the poolside or bottom at injury-producing speeds. Thus, off-axis dives are a foreseeable and necessary consideration in pool design if injury is to be avoided.

By using the length of the board for a running start, a person can achieve horizontal velocities ranging from 0 to 15 ft/s, (0 to 10.23 mi/h), depending on the length of the board and the nature of the run/jump. Photographic studies have shown that untrained divers, using a running approach, enter the water about 13 ft from the end of a 1-meter board; trained divers, using a correct approach and hurdle, enter at about 4 ft away from the board.

Stone[5] did the first in-depth mathematical treatment of diving mechanics. He has shown that an approximation for calculating the maximum distance from the end of the springboard to water entry for a dive is

$$D_{max} = 0.7 \ H + 4h_j + h_b$$

where H is the diver's height in feet, h_j is the maximum height the subject can jump in feet, and h_b is the height of the board above the water in feet. (The coefficient for h_j would be set equal to two for a platform dive.)

Gabrielsen[6] has shown that trained divers performing simple dives enter the water about 2 to 3 ft from the end of the board. Complicated dives by experts involving twists, turns, and somersaults result in entries up to 6 ft from the end of a 3-m board.

The higher the takeoff point is from the water, the farther out the entry point, unless a conscious effort is made by the diver to come close to the takeoff point. Photographic studies reveal that, from a takeoff point of 8 in. above the water, head entries up to 9 to 10 ft from the takeoff point are possible. Recreational divers, particularly youngsters, usually enter the water 4 to 6 ft from the takeoff point. From a running start, the athletic person can enter the water 12 to 15 ft from the pool edge.

WATER ENTRY SPEEDS

When executing a standing dive, the water entry speed of the diver's head varies by 3 to 5 ft/s depending on whether a near-vertical or a "flat" dive is performed. The head speed at entry is essentially the result of (1) initial takeoff velocity, (2) height of the springboard or platform above the water, and (3) diver's height. The near-vertical dive has a larger vertical-velocity component than the flat dive, and the flat dive has a larger horizontal-velocity component than the near-vertical dive. To better understand the magnitude associated with diving speeds, one can relate them to the speed of an object falling 12 in. At the end of the 12-in. fall, the object is moving at 8 ft/s (5.45 mi/h).

ANGLE OF ENTRY

The angle of entry can range from 0 degrees (belly flop) to greater than 90 degrees, depending on the takeoff flight and maximum height of the trajectory. The diver has the ability to achieve a steep water entry by jumping vertically or by jackknifing at the top of the trajectory, given either adequate takeoff height or proper training such as that necessary to perform the plain header decribed by Rackham[7]. To achieve a shallow entry, less than 30 degrees, the diver must lean forward on the takeoff. The so-called "racing dive" was always conceived as a flat dive with an entry angle of no more than 10 to 15 degrees. A current trend in racing dives, as exemplified by our best competitive swimmers, is to dive "into the hole." A break of the trunk at the maximum height of the above-water trajectory results in a clean entry (little splash) at about 45 degrees (see Figure 8.6). Immediately on immersion of the upper body, corrective action is taken to place the body in a more horizontal position by lifting the head and arching the back where planing forces then bring the swimmer to the surface.

For a clean dive from springboards and platforms very near the water surface, the water entry angle of the diver's upper torso is very nearly the same as the departure angle from the springboard or platform. As the height between the board or platform and the water increases, the angle of entry increases. When performing twists, somersaults, or other maneuvers, the diver can increase or decrease the entry configuration, resulting in increased hydrodynamic drag that causes a faster reduction of in-water speed and changes in the in-water trajectory.

In-Water Trajectory

Only after a significant portion of the diver's body (i.e., the upper torso) enters the water can the dive trajectory be appreciably altered. Until that time, the trajectory has been solely under the influence of gravitational attraction. However, as soon as effective water entry is achieved, these three new "forces" come into play:

- Net buoyancy
- Hydrodynamic drag
- Planing force (i.e., lift or other change in direction)

Stone,[8] using studies reported in DOT-T 90511a, has shown that a reasonable assumption can be made that the net buoyancy force is a small number. When small forces are compared with significantly larger forces, they can generally be ignored. Thus, in an analysis of the downward portion of the in-water trajectory of a dive, the net buoyancy force can be ignored.

Hydrodynamic drag force has the following form:

$$F = (1/2)\ C_d\ \rho A V^2$$

where F is the drag force, C_d is the coefficient of drag, ρ is the density of water A, is the body's cross-sectional area, and V is the in-water speed.

A clean dive (again, one in which the diver maintains alignment of the body with the trajectory of the center of mass) minimizes the effects of hydrodynamic drag. This results in higher speeds at a given depth and penetration to greater depths. Conversely, altering body alignment increases the drag force that then changes the in-water trajectory from that of a clean entry, resulting in lower speeds and shallower penetration depths. Based on various studies, the coefficient of drag for three-dimensional "bluff" bodies is essentially equal to one. According to Stone,[8] limited studies done on towed swimmers produced a range of 1.0 to 1.2 for the coefficient of drag.

Planing forces can be directed either upward or downward, depending on the body's angle of attack relative to the in-water trajectory. Body components such as the hands, arms, and upper trunk can be positioned to cause upward, downward, or sideward increased drag or rotational changes in direction. However, in the theoretical clean dive where the body is aligned with the trajectory, the planing force is zero.

The diver's in-water path is determined by actions taken after water entry. If the body alignment is straight with arms clamped tightly against the ears, the angle at water entry can be maintained quite easily. Factors that may affect the diver's in-water trajectory are raising or lowering of the head, altering the position of the arms, changing the attitude of the hands, arching the back, piking at the hips, and tucking in the legs. These movements not only change the diver's direction and body configurations but also slow in-water movement because of increased hydrodynamic drag. As a result, in analyzing the "worst-case" aspects of diving, the clean dive with entry angles greater than 30 degrees represents the most dangerous entry into shallow water.

IN-WATER SPEEDS

Based on photographic studies, in a clean dive hydrodynamic drag generally does not start to slow the diver's in-water speed to values less than that at water entry until a significant portion of the diver's body is immersed. On the order of one half to three fourths of the body must be in the water when executing a clean dive before deceleration commences. Research related to the adult-sized diver has shown that, after immersion, the speed of the body is halved for every 8 ft of travel through the water.

The speed of the diver in water is determined by entry speed, body alignment, and hydrodynamic drag. From the study of a 200 frames per second motion picture film of a diver (70 in. tall, weight 160 lb, diving from an elevation 8 in. above the water, a clean water-entry angle of approximately 45 degrees), the following head speeds were measured as shown in Table 10.1.

It is interesting to note that the diver's maximum in-water speed was not achieved until the top of the head reached a depth of 2.5 ft, or about 42 in. of the diver's body was immersed in the water. The speed of the diver's head was nearly the same at water entry as when about 55 in. of the diver's body was immersed. A grid, divided into 1×1 ft squares, was placed behind the diver, which permitted these measurements to be made.

IMPACT FORCES

Although in-water speeds may be great, they do not present a cause for concern unless the diver impacts a relatively immovable barrier. However, pools, lakes, rivers, etc. do have such barriers as represented by bottoms, sides, and objects. Head contact with these barriers or objects at sufficient speeds and angles can produce serious injury. In these instances, the old adage, "It was not the fall but the sudden stop," is true. When the motion of the diver's head is temporarily stopped, the torso, containing the center of mass, attempts to continue its motion. The bones in the neck are then compressively loaded and the resultant force can be sufficient to cause irreversible injuries (see Chapter 11). A good visualization of this process is the result when a freight train engine suddenly stops and the cars try to continue their motion through the stopped engine.

By assuming a diver makes head contact with the bottom or other barrier, the normal component (i.e., the component perpendicular to the barrier) of the velocity at contact is essentially brought instantaneously to zero. Actually this change occurs over the small fraction of time required for the body and the barrier material to slightly "give" or dissipate the energy of the impact. For a concrete pool bottom, this distance is on the order of 1 in.

TABLE 10.1
Head Speeds

Depth (ft)	Head Speed (ft/s)	Depth (ft)	Head Speed (ft/s)
0.5	14.0	3.5	12.8
1.0	14.4	4.0	11.2
1.5	14.9	4.5	9.7
2.0	15.3	5.0	8.4
2.5	15.7	5.5	7.2
3.0	14.3	6.0	7.0
		6.5	6.8

Compressive forces for a 175-lb diver impacting a hard bottom at speeds ranging from 0 to 12 ft/s and at angles ranging from 0 to 90 degrees can range from 0 to almost 4700 lb. Due to the spinal column being a linked apparatus, whether the head is neutrally aligned, flexed, or extended is of no concern because the compressive force is transmitted as though the head–neck system were in alignment. However, in terms of the force required to cause onset of injury, the position of the head is important because less of the surface area of a vertebral body is used to absorb the compressive force in flexion and extension as compared with neutral alignment. Thus, less force is needed to produce traumatic injury when the head is flexed or extended.

As the torso angle of impact and/or speed increases, the compressive loading on the head–neck system dramatically increases. Forces on the order of 100 to 1000 lb are sufficient to cause quadriplegic injuries, depending on the relationship of the head to the neck. According to Kazarian, the threshold force for fracturing the skull due to head impact is on the order of 1700 lb.

The larger the vertical component of the velocity vector (i.e., the greater the torso impact angle), the greater the compressive loading on the spine. This is what makes diving beyond the well, or the deep portion of residential or motel/hotel pools, so dangerous. When entering the water far out from the end of the springboard or platform, head contact can be made with the upslope section of the pool bottom. The slope section is the region where the transition from deep water to shallow water occurs. Even though a clean dive with a water entry angle of only 30 degrees may be executed, if the slope has a one-in-three rise, then head contact with the slope could occur at near 50 degrees relative to the slope. A larger vertical component of the velocity vector, resulting in a larger compressive force on the spinal column, results if the arms and hands do not deflect the trajectory.

MATHEMATICAL MODELING OF DIVING INJURIES

Although it is not possible to reconstruct a diving accident, simulation using a computer model can reveal the range of values most likely to be associated with various diving parameters. The computer model uses equations and techniques that have been in existence for several hundred years.

HORIZONTAL EQUATIONS

The equations for locating the horizontal position, x, of some reference point and for determining the horizontal velocity, V_x, at some time, given no accelerated motion in the horizontal direction, for a body undergoing motion in the $x - y$ plane are

$$x = x_0 + V_{x0}t \tag{1}$$

and

$$V_x = V_{x0} \tag{2}$$

where x_0 is the reference points initial x location, V_{x0} is the initial horizontal velocity, and t is time.

In analyzing diving trajectories, the initial takeoff speed, V_0, is determined by the leg and arm thrust, plus the throw of a springboard, if used. Consider for the moment that, in diving from the edge of a pool or a platform, only the thrust generated by leg and arm movements is involved. From energy conservation principles, this initial speed can be calculated by determining the height an individual can reach in performing a standing jump. By equating the jumper's kinetic energy to the potential energy, one can solve for the initial speed at takeoff. Because

$$2\,mgh = mV_0^2 \tag{3}$$

then

$$V_0 = (2\,gh)^{1/2} \tag{4}$$

where g is gravitational acceleration, and h is the height jumped vertically.

Given this initial speed, V_0, plus a take-off angle, Θ_0, measured relative to the horizontal, and assuming that the diver's center of mass, cm, is located at one half of the diver's height, H, then the x-coordinate of the location of the diver's cm at some time, t, measured relative to the takeoff point, can be calculated from

$$X_{cm} = (H/2 + V_0 t)\cos\Theta_0 \tag{5}$$

Vertical Equations

The equations for locating the vertical position, y, of some reference point, and for determining the vertical velocity, V_y, at some time, given accelerated motion in the vertical direction, for a body undergoing motion in the $x - y$ plane are

$$Y = y_0 + V_{y0} t - gt^2/2 \tag{6}$$

and

$$V_y = V_{y0} - gt \tag{7}$$

where y_0 is the reference point's initial y-location, and V_{y0} is the initial vertical velocity.

For the diving analysis, the y-coordinate of the location of the center of mass, measured relative to the surface of the water, requires the addition of the height of the takeoff point above the water surface to Equation (6). Thus

$$y_{cm} = (H/2 + V_0 t)\sin\Theta_0 - gt^2/2 + h_w \tag{8}$$

where h_w is the height of takeoff point above water.

By eliminating time between Equations (5) and (8), y can be related to x using

$$y_{cm} = x_{cm}\tan\Theta_0 - g\,((x_{cm} - H\cos\Theta_0/2)/2\,V_0\cos\Theta_0)^2 + h_w \tag{9}$$

Water-Entry Angle and Head Speed

This analysis assumes that the diver makes a clean dive. Such a dive has the major portions of the body aligned with the trajectory of the center of mass. This results in a clean water entry (i.e., one in which there is minimum cross-sectional area and, as a result, minimum hydrodynamic drag).

By the time the diver's head reaches the surface of the water, assuming a normal dive with arms and hands extended, the equations governing free fall no longer apply because of the resistance of water. While in the air, and at heights of less than 50 ft, the resistance of air can be ignored. Water, however, is over 800 times more dense than air and its resistance cannot be ignored. To calculate the body's in-water speed, the speed of the diver's head at water entry must be calculated first.

The time of flight from takeoff until head contact with the water's surface, neglecting hand and arm effects, if any, can be solved using

$$(H/2 + V_0 t)\sin\Theta_0 - gt^2/2 + h_w + H\sin\Theta_w/2 = 0 \tag{10}$$

where Θ_w is the water-entry angle at head contact.

The water-entry angle, Θ_w, can be solved from

$$\Theta_w = \tan^{-1}((V_0 \sin\Theta_0 - gt)/V_0 \cos\Theta_0) \qquad (11)$$

Now, Equations (10) and (11) can be solved in a simultaneous manner or by using iteration techniques on a computer. The solution for time permits the calculation of the vertical velocity of the diver's head at water entry, V_{yw}, using Equation (7). The speed of the head at water entry, V_w, then can be calculated using

$$V_w = (V_0 \cos\Theta_0^2 + V_{yw}^2)^{1/2} \qquad (12)$$

IN-WATER HEAD SPEED

Once in the water, the diver's body can take any number of paths, depending on how the diver positions the major portions of the body relative to the trajectory of the center of mass. This analysis is concerned with maintaining a clean path in water, and thus determining maximum speed at any depth as a result of minimum hydrodynamic drag. A useful equation for such analysis has been shown to be of the form

$$V_d = V_w e^{-C(p - fH)} \qquad (13)$$

where V_d is the head velocity at depth d; C is the coefficient, a function of the diver's height; p is the path length in water to get to depth d; and f is a fraction (nominally 0.5 to 0.7).

A delay fraction, f, is used based on high-speed motion picture analyses. After water entry, the speed of the diver's head continues to increase for a short duration during a clean dive because hydrodynamic drag does not begin to slow the diver down immediately. Generally, the diver's head speed does not slow down to equal the speed at water entry until after the center of mass enters the water. Thus, a value of 0.5 to 0.7 is normally used to account for this observation in that the center of mass is nominally located at approximately one half of the diver's height. It has been shown that C can be set equal to the coefficient of drag for bluff bodies, 1.1, divided by twice the diver's height, with good results for clean dives.

INTRODUCTION TO THE WORK–ENERGY THEOREM

The need to relate cervical X-rays to the mechanics of motion involving head impact with a hard object is frequently encountered in aquatic accidents involving traumatic spinal cord injuries (i.e., broken necks). Of particular interest are the compressive forces needed to cause the injuries and the velocities at impact.

Before going further, an understanding of the difference between speed and velocity is needed. Speed is a scalar quantity. A scalar quantity possesses magnitude only and not direction. For example, information that a car is being driven at an average speed of 30 mi/h only conveys knowledge concerning how fast the car is moving. If additional information is provided that the car is also heading east at this average speed, then not only how fast the car is traveling but also the direction is known. When both magnitude and direction are given, one is dealing with a vector quantity. If motion of a body is involved, this vector quantity is called velocity. (In addition to the need to have magnitude and direction, a vector must also obey the laws of vector addition.)

Force is another example of a quantity that satisfies vector requirements just as velocity does. However, force does not exist on its own account. It is instead a concept. The efforts of Isaac Newton (1642 to 1727) first gave us the ability to deal with this concept when he formulated his laws of motion, particularly his second law. This fundamental law of classical mechanics states that the acceleration (also a vector) of some mass is equal to the vector sum of all forces acting on that mass, divided by the mass itself.

Notice, however, that a new term, mass, has been introduced into the discussion involving force. What is mass? First, let us talk about weight, for example, your weight. Your weight is the result of the gravitational attraction of the earth. Your weight is a vector quantity, a vector force. The direction is toward the center of the earth and the magnitude is expressed in force units, such as pounds or newtons. By using Newton's second law, $F = ma$, the definition of mass is made. It is the result of dividing your weight by the magnitude of the gravitational attraction. While it is true that your weight changes in different locations on the earth because the magnitude of the gravitational attraction changes from locale to locale, your mass or, for that matter, the mass of any other object does not change. Mass is known as an intrinsic property of a body. For example, although in space flight in a "zero g" environment you would be weightless, nevertheless, your body would still have form and substance and thus mass. The same, identical force is required to cause a given acceleration in gravity-free space as in a frictionless environment on the earth. Mass can be thought of as the measure of a body's inertia or resistance to being moved. Using English units of measurement, the mass of a body is given in "slugs." If a body weighs 161 lb on the earth and the magnitude of gravitational acceleration is 32.2 ft/s^2, then the mass of that body is 5 slugs.

Of particular importance concerning Newton's second law, $F = ma$, is that this law is only a theory. It cannot be proved from first principles. This law exists because numerous observations consistently produce the same results over and over again. $F = ma$ is accepted because it works. If someone should ever come along and be able to show just one example where it does not work, then the whole of classical mechanics would be cast into utter disarray and the entire concept of physics would have to be recast.

Calculations associated with an impact against a hard object can be addressed using the work–energy theorem. Because the concept relating work and energy is based on Newton's second law, which is a theory, then it likewise is a theory. The same comments apply concerning its believability.

In physics, the concept of work is defined as the amount of force required to move a body some distance or displacement. Work is a scalar (i.e., it only has magnitude). However, both force and displacement are vectors. This is an extremely important finding. Work is only done when a force acts in the same direction or in an opposite direction to the displacement. The vertical force holding a body at some fixed distance above the ground does no work on the body, even if the body is moved horizontally. (Keep in mind that a physics concept is being addressed here.) If the trigonometric relationship involving the cosine of the angle between the force vector and the displacement vector is not included when making a calculation using the work–energy theorem, then one gets a wrong answer. The use of the cosine function is what converts the product of two vectors, force and displacement, into a scalar. Why is that important?

As one might guess, the work–energy theorem relates the amount of work required to cause a change in a body's energy. Energy is also a scalar (i.e., it only has magnitude). If an equation is to be true, then what is on the left side must equal what is on the right side. Otherwise, one would be trying to deal with apples and oranges. Because energy is a scalar, work also must be a scalar.

What is energy? Of interest is the concept of kinetic energy or the energy of motion. In physics, the kinetic energy of a body is defined as one half of the product of the body's mass and the square of the body's speed. (Note that the use of speed is what makes kinetic energy a scalar.) The work done on a body by a resultant force is always equal to the change in the kinetic energy of the body. (A resultant force is nothing more than the vector sum of all the forces acting on a body.)

Thus, we have arrived at the concept of the work–energy theorem. The equation is

$$Fd\cos\Theta = m(S_f^2 - S_i^2)/2 \qquad (14)$$

where F = force in pounds, d = displacement in feet, Θ = angle between F and d, m = mass in slugs, S_f = final speed in feet per second, and S_i = initial speed in feet per second.

Given that a change in a body's speed can be measured and the distance over which the change occurs is also known, then the force needed to cause a change in the body's kinetic energy can be calculated. The theorem has four variables. These are force, displacement, mass, and speed. Therefore, given sufficient information about three of these four variables, calculations of the unknown variable can be accomplished.

However, to apply the theorem to calculations involving impacts with relatively immovable barriers such as a head impact with a swimming pool or lake bottom, an additional consideration must be made. Of interest is the force exerted on the body at the moment of impact when the body can no longer go through the barrier as a result of contact. In other words, the approach velocity component perpendicular to the barrier is abruptly changed to zero. Note that although what happens to the body after initial impact with the barrier may be of importance to some other question, it is of no importance when calculating the force at initial contact that reduces the perpendicular velocity component to zero.

This is the point where the finding becomes extremely important. From studies based on engineering mechanics, a barrier can only exert a force in a direction perpendicular to the barrier. For example, when an object is at rest on a horizontal floor, the floor exerts a force perpendicular to the floor in opposition to the weight of the object. Because work is a scalar, only the displacement in the same direction or in the opposite direction to the force can be used when work–energy theorem calculations are made. Any other approach produces the wrong answer.

For instance, given the speed and the angle of the upper torso at impact, the weight of the diver, and an assumption concerning the displacement, the average spinal compressive force caused by the "sudden stop" (i.e., reduction of the perpendicular component of the impact velocity to zero, due to contacting a relatively immovable barrier) can be calculated from

$$F = W(S_i \sin\Theta_i)^2/2\,gd \tag{15}$$

where F = average compressive force in pounds, W = diver's weight in pounds, S_i = impact speed in feet per second, Θ_i = impact angle in degrees, g = 32.2 ft/s^2, and d = displacement in feet. Given that an impact of the sort being described here occurs over a very short time period, the peak compressive force exerted on the spine is simply twice the average force.

Let us suppose a 161-lb diver impacts the bottom at 10 ft/s at an angle of 30 degrees. Assuming a displacement of 1 in., what is the peak compressive force exerted on the diver's body? If you do not get 1500 lb, try again.

Now suppose that the peak compressive force exerted on the 161-lb diver's body at impact is 800 lb. Given a contact speed of 10 ft/s and assuming a displacement of 1 in., what is the impact angle of the upper torso?

If you do not get approximately 21.4 degrees, try again.

SIMULATION ANALYSES

Various computer simulations using a diver 6 ft 0 in. (72 in.) tall and weighing 175 lb have been run. Significant results are presented in the following sections.

DIVES FROM 6-IN. DECK

Assume that two divers, one below average and one above average in athletic abilities, are performing a standing, clean dive from a deck that is 6 in. above the water surface. Significant results for a racing or shallow-type dive (i.e., takeoff angles on the order of 10 to 40 degrees above the horizontal) are

Distance to head entry (ft)	6.81–9.32
Water entry speed (ft/s)	8.64–13.79
Water entry angle (degrees)	21.57–55.56
Time of flight (s)	0.15–0.56
Speed at 3.0-ft depth (ft/s)	6.41–14.22

DIVES FROM $^1/_2$ M

Diving from 1/2 m using the board and using takeoff angles ranging from 40 to 70 degrees above the horizontal produces the following ranges for the below-average and above-average divers:

Distance to head entry (ft)	5.09–14.10
Water entry speed (ft/s)	15.94–20.79
Water entry angle (degrees)	51.57–77.09
Time of flight (s)	0.64–1.09
Speed at 3.0-ft depth (ft/s)	9.24–13.62

DIVES FROM 1 M

Diving from 1 m using the board and making the same dives produces the following ranges for the below-average and above-average divers:

Distance to head entry (ft)	5.36–15.05
Water entry speed (ft/s)	18.77–23.16
Water entry angle (degrees)	56.24–78.90
Time of flight (s)	0.74–1.17
Speed at 3.0-ft depth (ft/s)	9.80–13.25

CONCLUSIONS

The analyses leave one with an inescapable conclusion. Divers must be given an adequate volume of water in which to finish their dives and maneuver to return safely to the water's surface. If an adequate water volume for safe diving or headfirst sliding cannot be provided, then the body of water may be suitable for swimming only. If so, then adequate warnings must be posted prohibiting diving and headfirst slides (see Chapter 13).

ACKNOWLEDGMENT

The analyses in this chapter based on physics and computer simulations were contributed by Dr. George E. T. Lawniczak, Jr.

REFERENCES

1. Gerrish, W., A Dynamic Analysis of the Standing Vertical Jump, Doctoral Dissertation, Teacher's College, Columbia University, New York, 1934.
2. Considine, W. S. and Sullivan, E. J., Relationship of selected tests of leg strength and leg power on college men, *Res. Q.*, 44.4, 404, December 1974.

3. Offenbacher, E. J., Physics and the vertical jump, *Am. J. Phys.,* 38, 829, 1969.
4. Batterman, C., *The Techniques of Springboard Diving,* MIT Press, Cambridge, MA, 1968.
5. Stone, R. S., Diving Safety in Swimming Pools: A Report to the National Swimming Pool Foundation, Arthur D. Little, Cambridge, MA, May 1980.
6. Gabrielsen, M. A., *Photographic Analysis of Underwater Action of International Diving Champions,* Consumer Product Safety Commission (CPSC), Washington, D.C., 1975.
7. Rackman, G., *Diving Complete,* Faber & Faber, London, United Kingdom, 1975.
8. Stone, R. S., Buoyancy and Stability Characteristics of the Human Body in Fresh Water, Final Report, On Contract DO7-CG 90511a, U.S. Coast Guard, November 1971.

11 Biomechanical Aspects of Cervical Trauma from Diving

INTRODUCTION

From a mechanical and structural point of view, the cervical spine is a very complex mechanism. The human neck contains vital neurological, vascular, and respiratory structures as well as the cervical vertebrae and spinal cord. Although injury statistics generally attribute only 2 to 4% of serious trauma to the neck, any neck injury can have debilitating if not life-threatening consequences. Permanent paralysis is a particularly devastating and costly injury. When it is a consequence of accidental trauma, frequently a young productive member of society is transformed into a totally dependent member. The advent of high-speed land and air transportation has made us increasingly aware of the serious consequences that can result from a structural failure of the neck. Also, as more people pursue leisure-time activities, the potential for serious neck injuries increases. Football, diving, gymnastics, skiing, hang gliding, mountain climbing, and amusement rides are but a few activities that expose the neck to a risk of serious injury. As a result, a variety of devices have evolved that offer a measure of protection to the neck from mechanical trauma. Head and seat restraints, motorcycle and football helmets, energy-absorbing pads and collars, and gymnastic mats are but a few examples of head and neck protective devices. Unfortunately, the design of many of these has proceeded with insufficient biomechanical input because of the lack of relevant data. Fortunately, because of increased federal funding, the amount of available information on neck injuries has increased dramatically in the last decade. This chapter summarizes research aimed at providing some biomechanical responses of the neck in a form that is useful in understanding cervical injury mechanisms and in development of societal strategies to reduce the number of cervical spine injuries. To that end, various biomechanical characteristics of the neck, tolerance criteria, and injury mechanisms are presented.

INCIDENCE

The National Head and Spinal Cord Injury Survey estimated the occurrence of spinal cord injury with quadriplegia in the United States at 5 per 100,000 or in excess of 10,000 new cases each year. According to the National Spinal Cord Injury Database, which catalogs data from approximately 15% of these new cases, cervical lesions were documented in 51% of discharged patients with 39.5% occurring in the lower cervical spine: 12.9% at C-4, 14.9% at C-5, and 11.7% at C-6.[1] Despite the relative low frequency of these injuries, the large direct medical costs and lost productivity result in annual costs that are conservatively estimated at $97 billion.[2]

While injuries to the cervical spine can result from almost any activity, the literature suggests that automobile accidents, sports, gunshot wounds, and falls are the circumstances most often identified (Table 11.1). Unfortunately, injuries due to violence (mainly gunshot wounds) have increased dramatically over the last two decades.[1]

TABLE 11.1
Activity Associated with Cervical Spinal Cord Injury

	Reported Cases	
Category	Number	Percentage
Auto accident	842	36.7
Fall	365	15.9
Gunshot wound	268	11.7
Shallow water diving	243	10.6
Motorcycle accident	143	6.2
Hit by falling/flying object	124	5.4
Other	61	2.7
Other sports	60	2.6
Football	29	1.3
Pedestrian	29	1.3
Medical/surgical complication	28	1.2
Bicycle	22	1.0
Other vehicular	19	0.8
Fixed-wing aircraft	7	0.3
Trampoline	15	0.7
Stabbing	9	0.4
Rotating-wing aircraft	7	0.3
Snow skiing	6	0.3
Snowmobile	5	0.2
Water skiing	4	0.2
Unknown	4	0.2
Boat	2	0.1
Total	2292	

Data from the National Spinal Cord Injury Data Research Center (NSCIDRC), University of Alabama at Birmingham, April 1999. with permission.

TABLE 11.2
Cause and Severity of Spinal Fractures in Canada (1980–1986)

Cause of Injury	Total (N)	Injuries (%)
Motor vehicle accident	768	53
Occupational	221	15
Domestic	203	14
Sporting and recreational	202	14
Other	54	4
Total	1448	

Adapted from Allen, D. G., Reid, D. C., and Saboe, L., 1988. with permission.

The distribution of injuries depends somewhat on the location of the data collection as is evidenced by the comparison of Table 11.1 with the Canadian experience (Table 11.2[3]). However, the general trends are similar.

Sports and leisure activities account for a significant portion of injuries to the cervical spine. In 1978, Shield, et al.[4] analyzed 10 years of data on 152 cervical spinal cord injuries caused by sports participation that were treated at the Rancho Los Amigos Hospital (Table 11.3). Considerable

TABLE 11.3
Sport Activity Causing Cervical Spinal Cord Damage in 152 Individuals

Activity	Number	Percent
Diving	82	54
Football	16	11
Gymnastics	5	3
Snow skiing	5	3
Surfing	29	19
Track and field	3	2
Trampoline	2	1
Water skiing	7	5
Wrestling	3	2
Total	152	

From Shield, L. K., Fox, B., and Stauffer, E. S. (1978). *Physician sports Med.*, 6, 321, 1978. with permission.

TABLE 11.4
Spine Injuries in Specific Sports

Diving	43	21.3
Snowmobiles[a]	20	9.9
Parachute/skydiving	20	9.9
Equestrian	19	9.4
Dirt bikes	18	8.9
All-terrain vehicle	15	7.4
Toboggan[a]	11	5.4
Alpine skiing[a]	11	5.4
Ice hockey[a]	6	3.0
Rugby	6	3.0
Bicycle	5	2.5
Football	4	2.0
Wrestling	3	1.5
Mountaineering	3	1.5
Surfing	3	1.5
Other	15	7.4
Total	202	

Adapted from Reid, D. C. and Saboe, L., *Sports Med.*, 7(6), 393, 1989. with permission.

[a] Winter sports: 48 Injuries (24%).

regional variation in sports-related cervical injury exists primarily due to the degree of participation in the various activities. However, these injuries can be generally classified as most commonly resulting from contact sports (of which football is the most well known) and falls and dives from a height. The incidence of cervical injuries in the game of football is described by Torg[5] and Torg et al.[6–8] using the National Football Injury Register.

Swimming and diving accidents have also been identified as causing significant numbers of fractures and dislocations of the cervical spine. Kewalramani and Taylor[9] found that 18% of all spinal cord injuries in their series of cases were related to diving accidents. Albrand and Walter[10] published curves that related depth in feet and head velocity to the height of the diver above the water. McElhaney et al.[11] also provided experimental data relative to body velocity and depth of the water. This series of accidents included not only springboard diving but also water slides (an early work on water slides is by Gabrielsen and McElhaney[12]). McElhaney et al.[11] suggested that a head velocity of approximately 10 ft/s (3.05 m/s) with a following body is sufficient to cause compression fractures of the cervical spine, most frequently at the level of C-5, the fifth cervical vertebra. As this is equivalent to a vertical drop height of only 19.4 in., we realize that many activities, including the activities of daily living, contain the potential for neck injury. Reid and Saboe[13] provide a proportionate distribution of such injuries in specific sports (Table 11.4). Care must be exercised in interpreting data of these types because the incidence is determined more by the number of participants and exposures than by other factors.

ANATOMY

The complete spine is a structure composed of 7 cervical, 12 thoracic, 5 lumbar, 5 sacral, and 4 coccygeal vertebrae. Each vertebra is composed of a cylindrical vertebral body connected to a series of bony elements collectively referred to as the posterior elements. The posterior elements include the pedicles, the lamina, the spinous and the transverse processes, and the superior and inferior facet joint surfaces. This structure is also known as the neural arch. It provides mechanical protection for the spinal cord and contributes to the stability and kinematics of the vertebral column.

The cervical spine is comprised of seven vertebrae, which form eight motion segments between the base of the skull and the first thoracic vertebra, T-1 (Figure 11.1). The vertebrae are numbered so that the uppermost vertebra is denoted C-1, also called the atlas; and the lowermost vertebra is C-7. The motion segments are similarly labeled C-1 through C-8. C-1 denotes the articulation of the base of the skull with the first cervical vertebra, and C-8 denotes the articulation of the C-7 vertebra with T-1. Because this nomenclature scheme gives an identical name to the motion segment superior to the vertebra of the same name (e.g., motion segment C-4 is superior to the C-4 vertebra), an alternate labeling scheme is often used for clarification. The motion segment and intervertebral disk between two vertebrae can be described with reference to both surrounding vertebrae. For example, the C-4 motion segment is also called the C-3 to C-4 motion segment. These vertebrae and motion segments can be structurally grouped because the cervical spine is divided morphologically and mechanically into two regions, the upper cervical and lower cervical spine.

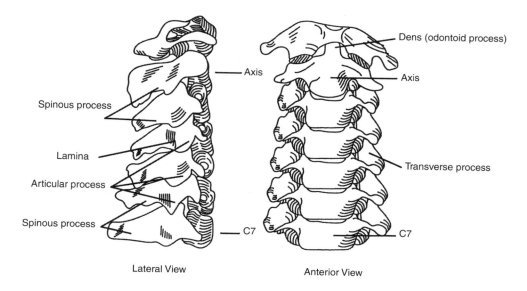

Lateral View   Anterior View

FIGURE 11.1 Lateral and anterior views of the bony cervical vertebrae.

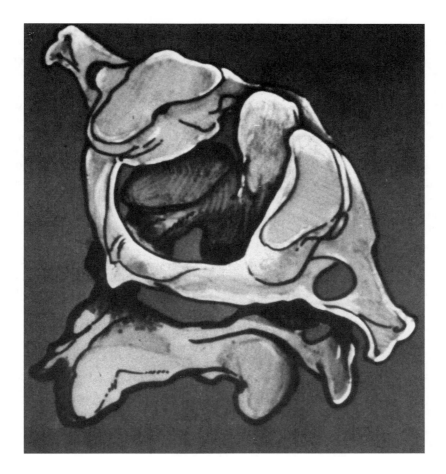

FIGURE 11.2 Bony anatomy of the first two cervical vertebrae, atlas, and axis.

The upper cervical spine consists of three bony elements: the occiput (the base of the skull), the atlas (C-1), and the axis (C-2). They produce two joints—the occipitoatlantal joint (C-1 or occiput-C-1) and the atlantoaxial joint (C-2 or C-1, 2) (Figure 11.2). The atlas is a bony ring, as it has no vertebral body unlike the other vertebrae, with enlarged facets on the lateral portions of the ring. The atlas is divided into the anterior and posterior arches. The anterior arch forms a synovial articulation with the second cervical vertebra, the axis, and the posterior arch provides protection for the spinal column and brain stem. The axis is composed of a vertebral body and a posterior bony arch, like the vertebrae in the lower cervical spine, but it has an additional element, the odontoid process (the dens). The odontoid process points superiorly from the C-2 vertebral body, and its anterior surface articulates with the posterior portion of the anterior arch of the atlas. The lateral portions of the axis contain flattened, enlarged articular facet surfaces; and lateral to these surfaces are the transverse processes.

The occipitoatlantal joint, which allows flexion–extension rotation, is formed by two bony protuberances, the occipital condylus, on the base of the skull and the atlas. The atlantoaxial joint, which allows axial head rotation, is composed of three synovial articulations between the atlas and the axis. The superior facet surfaces of the axis form two synovial articulations with the inferior facet surfaces of the atlas. The other synovial joint is formed by the articulation of the anterior arch of the atlas with the odontoid process of the axis.

The ligamentous structures of the occipitoatlantoaxial complex include continuations of the lower cervical ligaments and an additional set of structures unique to the upper cervical spine. The transverse ligament is a stout horizontal ligament that connects the medial portions of the C-1 lateral masses and constrains the odontoid process posteriorly. The transverse ligament is the horizontal portion of the cruciate ligament. The vertical portion of this ligament attaches to the anterior inferior aspect of foramen magnum of the base of the skull and the posterior aspect of the C-2 vertebral body. The apical ligament is a midline structure that connects the apex of the odontoid to the base of the skull anterior to the cruciate ligament. The alar ligaments originate on the posterior lateral aspect of the odontoid process and ascend laterally to insert directly to the base of the skull. The posterior longitudinal ligament inserts on the base of the skull posterior to the transverse ligament and is named the tectorial membrane. The anterior longitudinal ligament (ALL) inserts on the base of the skull. The anterior atlantoepistrophical and atlantooccipital ligaments lie posterior to the anterior longitudinal ligament and connect the C-2 vertebral body to the atlas and the atlas to the base of the skull, respectively. The lower cervical flaval ligaments insert on the base of the skull and are denoted the posterior atlantooccipital membrane. Finally, the nuchal ligament, which is formed by the midline fusion of the paravertebral muscular fascia, inserts on the occipital protuberance, which is small bump on the back of the head just above the neck.

The lower cervical spine contains vertebrae C-3 through C-7 and motion segments C-3 through C-8. The vertebrae, increasing in absolute size from superior to inferior, are geometrically similar with a cylindrical vertebral body and a posterior bony arch. The vertebral bodies are connected to

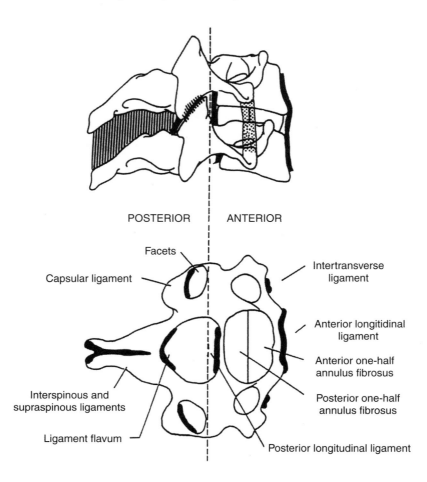

FIGURE 11.3 Schematic representation of the ligamentous anatomy of the cervical spine. (From White, A. A. and Panjabi, M. M., *Clinical Biomechanics of the Spine,* 2nd ed., Lippincott, Philadelphia, 1990 with permission.)

one another by a fibrocartilaginous intervertebral disk. This structure is composed of a central fluidlike nucleus pulposus bounded by a laminar set of spirally wound fibrous sheets denoted the annulus fibrosus. The anterior surfaces of the vertebral bodies are connected from the sacrum to the base of the skull by the anterior longitudinal ligament (Figure 11.3[14]). Similarly, the posterior longitudinal ligament connects the posterior surface of the vertebral bodies and forms the anterior surface of the spinal canal. The pedicles run posterolaterally from the posterior of the vertebral bodies and terminate in the pars interarticularis. The pars interarticularis denotes a bony region bounded superiorly by the superior facet surface, inferiorly by the inferior facet surface, laterally by the transverse process, and medially by the spinal canal. Lateral to these elements are the transverse processes, which contain the vertebral artery, the major blood supply for the brain stem, and the posterior portions of the brain. This artery is contained in the foramen transversarium of the transverse process. The laminae project posteromedially from the pars interarticularis and meet at the midline. The laminae form the posterior lateral surface of the spinal canal. Protruding from the midline fusion of the two laminae on each vertebra is the spinous process. The spinous processes are the palpable protuberances on the dorsal surface of the neck and back.

The interspinous and supraspinous ligaments connect the spinous processes of adjacent vertebra. The flaval, yellow ligaments similarly connect adjacent laminae from the sacrum to the base of the skull. The facet joints are formed by the inferior facet surface of the superior vertebrae and the superior facet surface of the inferior vertebrae. These are synovial joints, which are wrapped in a capsular ligament. The spinal canal of the vertebrae is the location of the spinal cord. Nerve roots exit between adjacent vertebrae through the intervertebral foramen. This foramen is composed of the inferior vertebral notch of the superior vertebrae and the superior vertebral notch of the inferior vertebrae.

INJURY MECHANISMS AND CLASSIFICATIONS

Because the study of cervical spine trauma has evolved from a wide variety of institutions and sources, several authors have attempted to classify the injuries so that there can be agreement as to what investigators are referring to when describing a particular injury. These include Babcock,[15] Melvin et al.,[16] Moffatt et al.,[17] Portnoy et al.,[18] Allen et al.,[19] White and Panjabi,[20] Dolen,[21] Harris et al.,[22] and Myers and Winkelstein.[23] The rationale for these classifications has included retrospective reviews of patient data, whole and segmental cadaveric experimentation, and retrospective evaluations of various known injury environments.[5,11,19,24] The following discussion and injury classification draw on all three methods in an attempt to bring the advantages of each to our understanding of injury.

Some of the confusion in understanding injury classification schemes has evolved from the nomenclature describing it. For example, flexion of the head may be produced by rotation of the head on the neck, or may be the result of anteroinferior translation of the head relative to the torso. The confusion is further compounded by the communication differences between the disciplines that study injuries (Figures 11.4 and 11.5). As an example, the term *extension* is properly defined in a clinical setting as a motion that brings the long axis of the distal portion of a joint parallel with the long axis of the proximal portion.[25] In the context of the cervical spine, extension refers to a posteroinferior motion of the head relative to the torso and is usually associated with rotation of the head and spine. In contrast, in engineering terms, extension refers to the elongation of a member along its long axis, the clinical equivalent of traction.

Injury classification is further complicated by the methods used to determine the mechanism. The global motion of the head relative to the torso may not be the same as regional motions of the cervical spine. For example, the observation of a flexion motion of the head relative to the torso may actually be concurrent with local (i.e., a single motion segment) extension in the cervical spine and may produce an extension injury. Further, small movements of the impact location or the initial position of the head (less than 1.0 cm) have been shown to change the injury from compression–flexion to compression–extension in cadaveric studies.[26,27] In addition, the observed motions of the

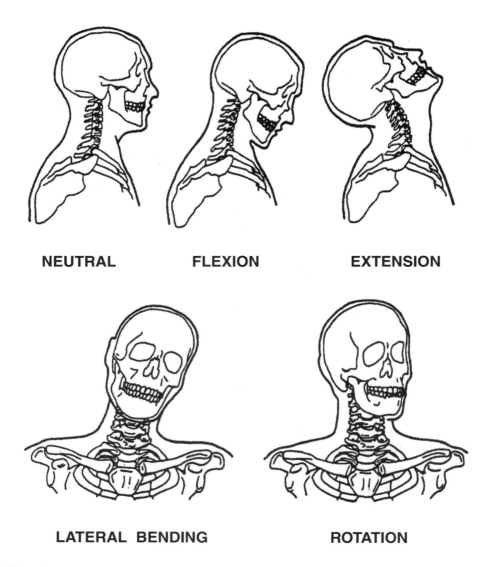

NEUTRAL   **FLEXION**   **EXTENSION**

LATERAL BENDING   **ROTATION**

FIGURE 11.4   Anatomic descriptions of head motion.

head may occur after the injury has occurred; thus, they may not reflect the true injury mechanism, but instead the motions of an unstable spine.[28] In this context, understanding whether the classifications are based on global motions of the head,[22] local deformations of the motion segment,[19] review of videotaped injuries, careful evaluation of patient data, or cadaveric experimentation is key to an understanding of injury classification.

COMPRESSION FRACTURES

COMPRESSION

Purely compressive loading of the cervical spine occurs infrequently due to the complexity of the cervical structure. Notwithstanding, many events may be considered to be predominantly vertical compressive loading. Cadaveric and clinical studies,[18,26,29–31] have demonstrated that axial displacement of the head can produce both upper and lower cervical compression injuries.

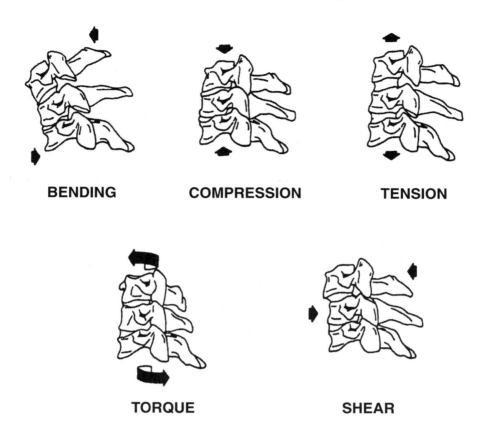

FIGURE 11.5 Engineering descriptions of neck loading.

Upper cervical compression injuries consist largely of multipart fractures of the atlas (Figure 11.6). While these fractures are frequently described as Jefferson fractures, the Jefferson fracture properly refers to a particular four-part fracture of the atlas.[32] Fatalities and instability from this group of injuries are common.[20] Basilar skull ring fractures, a fracture of the C-1 motion segment, are also the result of compressive loads.[31] Upper cervical injuries have also been reported with near vertex head impact testing, which resulted in alar ligament loading with sheer by the atlas and type III odontoid fractures.[34] While an odontoid fracture is likely a compression bending injury, to date the mechanism has yet to be reported.

Lower cervical vertebral body compression injuries occur at all vertebral levels from C-2 to T-1 (Figure 11.7). These lesions may consist of destruction of the cancellous bony centrum with loss of disk height, vertebral endplate fracture with vertical herniation of the nucleus pulposus into the centrum producing the so-called Schmorl's node, or multipart fractures of the vertebral body. The latter is referred to as a burst fracture (Figure 11.8). The most common sites of compression fractures in the lower cervical spine are C-4, C-5, and C-6[11] Ligamentous injury is relatively uncommon in pure vertical compression injuries, whereas damage to the facet joints and pars interarticularis commonly occurs. The risk of central neurological injury from these fractures is somewhat variable in the reported literature (approximately 40 to 75%), but tends to increase with the severity of the fracture.

COMPRESSION–FLEXION

Wedge compression fractures of the vertebral bodies are the result of a combination of a flexion bending moment and compressive loading of the vertebral motion segment resulting in greater

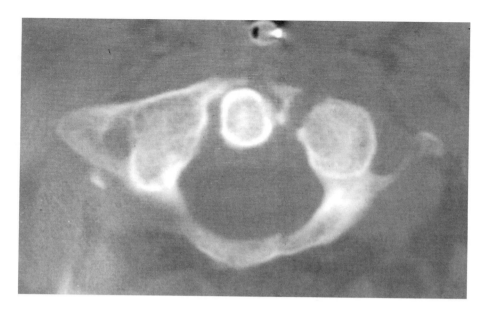

FIGURE 11.6 A computed tomography scan of a multipart atlas fracture, one of a variety of multipart fractures of the atlas that represent variations of the Jefferson fracture.

compressive stresses and failures in the anterior of the vertebral body. This type of injury is classified as compression–flexion and may be produced by compressive loading of the head, with or without actual head rotation. This has been demonstrated in cadaveric studies by McElhaney et al.[26] in which increasing the eccentricity (the effective moment arm of the applied axial load) during an axial displacement of the head produced wedge compression fractures, whereas decreased eccentricity of the applied loading produced compression and burst fractures (see Figure 11.8). Both of these types of fractures were produced in the absence of head rotation. These fractures usually occur in the lower three cervical segments where the flexible cervical spine joins the less flexible thorax, the flexion moments are the greatest, and the angular motion between vertebrae is the greatest.

A second group of injuries in the lower cervical spine has been classified clinically as both compressive hyperflexion[35] and distractive flexion (tension–flexion).[19,36] The former classification refers to blows occurring on the posterior portions of the head resulting in flexion of the head and compression of the spine. The latter classification refers to the presence of tensile stresses on the posterior elements and compressive loading on the vertebral body as a result of a flexion bending moment acting on the motion segment. As is discussed later, it would appear that both descriptions are accurate. This group of injuries includes unilateral facet dislocation, bilateral facet dislocation, and hyperflexion sprain.

Unilateral facet dislocation (UFD) refers to the anterosuperior displacement of a facet over the facet of the inferior vertebra with subsequent locking in a tooth-to-tooth fashion. In unilateral dislocation, the dislocation occurs in only one of the two facet joints of a motion segment. The most common sites of this injury are the C-5, C-6, and C-7 interspaces.[37] Clinically, the lesion is frequently asymptomatic or associated with radicular pain on the side of the injury (25 of 39 patients). Spinal cord injury is relatively uncommon in this type of injury, occurring in only 5 of 39 patients. The etiology of this lesion has been the subject of great interest and controversy. Huelke et al.[38] and Harris et al.[22] reported that unilateral dislocation was the result of combined flexion and rotation. Gosch et al.[39] reported that in purely anterior to posterior deceleration sled tests of primates, axial rotation was observed and unilateral facet dislocation was produced. Roaf[40] reported that torsion was required to produce lower cervical ligamentous injury and dislocation, and that

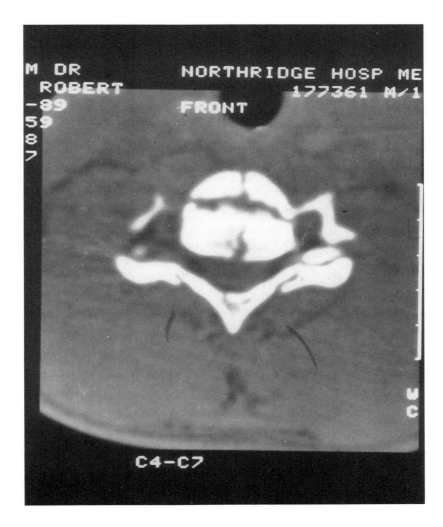

FIGURE 11.7   Cleavage fracture through the body and posterior arch.

hyperflexion alone could not produce ligamentous injury. Rogers[41] and White and Panjabi[20] noted that unilateral dislocation resulted from an exaggeration of the normal coupling of lower cervical lateral bending and rotation but did not describe the loads required to produce the injury. Braakman and Vinken[37] suggested that unilateral facet dislocation was the result of combined flexion and rotation. Torg[5] stated that the lesion was the result of compression and buckling. Bauze and Ardran[42] produced unilateral facet dislocations in a number of specimens loaded in compression and flexion. Their apparatus applied no torque to the specimen, and yet lower cervical rotation was observed prior to unilateral dislocation. Myers et al.[43] demonstrated that while unilateral facet dislocation could be produced by direct torsional loading of the lower cervical spine, the lesion could not be the result of torsional loading of the head because of the comparative weakness of the atlantoaxial joint. The authors currently believe that the lesion is produced by a mechanism similar to the bilateral facet dislocation with the difference being due to bending out of the plane of symmetry, or the presence of preexisting facet tropism of other structural asymmetry. As an additional note, facet dislocations are frequently referred to as fracture dislocations. This is because the apical portions of the facets are typically fractured or abraded during the injury when the flexion moment is the result of compressive loading.[22]

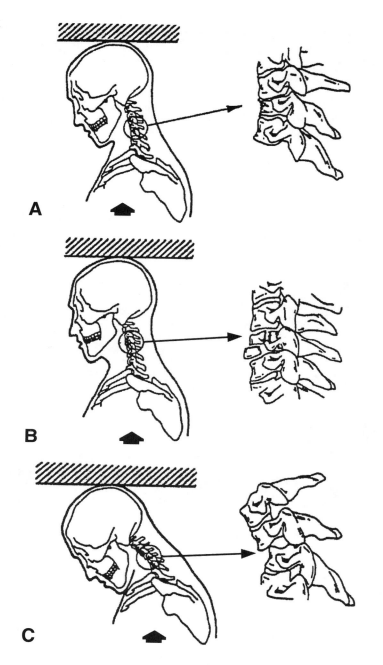

FIGURE 11.8 Schematic illustrating compression–flexion injury mechanisms. A. Wedge fracture. B. Burst fracture. C. Bilateral facet dislocation. The figure illustrates head rotation as part of the injury mechanism; however, research has shown that head rotation does not need to accompany this injury.

Bilateral facet dislocation (BFD) describes an injury in which the superior vertebral body is displaced anteriorly over its subjacent vertebra. This displacement results in a dislocation of both facet joints with subsequent locking of the surfaces in a tooth-to-tooth fashion secondary to muscle spasm. The lesion is more common in the lowest cervical motion segments; however, it can occur throughout the lower cervical spine.[19] Unfortunately, this injury results in greater than 50% anterolisthesis and significant reduction in the anteroposterior diameter of the neural canal, therefore usually being associated with spinal cord injury. Braakman and Vinken[37] report permanent, partial, or complete spinal cord injury in 27 of 35 patients with bilateral dislocations. Experimentally the lesion has been produced by Bauze and Ardran[42] and subsequently by Myers et al.[43] by applying a compressive axial displacement to cervical spines in which unconstrained posteroanterior displacement was permitted; however, rotation of the head was constrained. Analysis of load cell data from these experiments shows that the lower cervical spine was in a state of combined compression and flexion, and analysis of local deformations reveals the presence of tensile strains in the posterior ligaments prior to dislocation. Eccentricities of the applied forces as large as 7 cm were recorded. Evaluation and reconstruction of injury case histories suggest that loading of the head occurs more frequently in compression–flexion than in tension–flexion;[24] however, it also suggests that both types of loading may produce facet dislocations. Based on this observation it would appear that the primary injury vector is a lower cervical bending moment that is the result of a tensile or compressive eccentric load.

Hyperflexion sprain is a clinical entity in which the ligamentous structures of the posterior arch are torn or stretched without producing dislocations or fractures of the facet joints. It is thought to be produced by the same mechanism as bilateral facet dislocation, only with a less extensive disruption of the motion segment.[19] Harris et al.[22] report 30 to 50% of patients with this diagnosis develop late instability as a result of the ligamentous injury. Allen et al.[19] note that 2 of 12 patients with this diagnosis had spinal cord syndromes. It has been hypothesized based on these data that the hyperflexion sprain may represent a similar degree of injury as the other dislocations, with a spontaneous reduction of the dislocation at the time of injury.

COMPRESSION–EXTENSION

Extension can produce both lower and upper cervical injuries. The type of injury produced by extension bending moments (i.e., anterior ligamentous injury vs. posterior bony injury) depends largely on the type of head loading that produced the extension moment. These include anteroposterior shearing force (horizontal shear), compressive force directed posterior to the occipital condylus (compression–extension), and tensile forces with a line of action anterior to the occipital condylus (tension–extension). Local extension injuries may also occur in the presence of a flexion motion of the head relative to the torso. The effect of pure extension moment on cervical injury has not been investigated in a dynamic study because this type of loading is not likely to occur in the accident environment. Extension loading that produces structural damage to the lower cervical spine is less common than flexion injuries. The reasons for this may include the increased flexibility of the neck in extension over flexion, which allows the head to move out of the load path of the torso more easily; a decrease in the incidence of blows to the face as opposed to the crown and posterior of the head; or more likely the natural lordosis of the cervical spine that results in forward angulation of the neck relative to the head.

Compression–extension loading produces fractures of the posterior elements of the cervical spine. This has been observed in both clinical studies and experimental studies on the cadaveric specimens.[19,26,30,31,45] These injuries occur throughout the upper and lower cervical spine and appear to be the result of direct bony impingement of the posterior bony elements against each other. They also occur in conjunction with burst fractures. The types of injuries produced naturally depend on the relative magnitudes of the compression force and extension bending moments. These include laminar fractures, pedicle fractures, crushing injuries of the pars interarticularis, and fractures of the spinous processes. These fractures can occur in isolation, but are frequently multiple. They may also be associated with neurological deficit as a result of impingement on the spinal cord by the bony or ligamentous fragments, or as a result of cord compromise from spondylolisthesis of the unstable spine. It has been suggested, but not shown experimentally, that the larger the component of compression relative to the extension moment is, the greater the likelihood of pars interarticularis fractures instead of posterior element fractures (i.e., laminar fractures). While there are many other cervical injury mechanisms, such as tension and torsion, they seldom occur in diving accidents and are not discussed here. For a more complete review of injury mechanisms see Nahm and Melvin.[46]

DIVING

A multidisciplinary team led by Gabrielsen,[47] studied 486 diving injuries. Of this number, 360 (74.1%) occurred in pools and 126(25.9%) occurred in a natural environment. The pool-related injuries included 76(21.1%) from dives from springboards, 194(53.9%) from dives into inground pools, and 92(25.6%) into aboveground pools. The most frequent site of injury was C-5 and C-5, 6 with 219(60.8%) of the injuries occurring at those locations. These injuries were predominantly compression–flexion injuries.

It is remarkable how few skull fractures and brain injuries occur in diving even though in many of these accidents the head strikes a concrete pool bottom. It is also noteworthy to consider the number of dives made into swimming pools that lead to these injuries. There are approximately 7 million swimming pools in the United States. In 1989, the U. S. Consumer Product Safety Commission (CPSC) summarized the diving problem as approximately 700 spinal cord diving injuries being estimated to occur in the United States annually as a result of recreational diving into residential and public pools, and other bodies of water. It has been further estimated that there are approximately 200,000 people presently living in the United States who have suffered traumatic spinal cord injuries and that diving may account for 9 to 10% of them. The mean life expectancy for these spinal cord injury victims is estimated at 30.2 years.

Spinal cord injuries (SCIs) from all types of sports represent 14.2% of the annual total SCIs (7900 total survivors). Recreational diving is estimated at 54 to 66% of these, which is nearly twice as much as all other sports combined including football, surfing, gymnastics, skiing, trampoline, horseback riding, etc. The National Swimming Pool Foundation (NSPF) states that nine out of ten diving injuries occur in 6 ft of water or less. The conclusion is that only a very small fraction of dives result in a serious cervical injury. However, there are a very great number of dives made each year and therefore a significant number of catastrophic injuries. It has been estimated that approximately half of diving injuries occur in rivers, lakes, and oceans. The distribution of the injury level in these dives shows a similar clustering at the C-5 and C-5, 6 levels.[47]

Diving injuries in rivers, lakes, and oceans typically involve fewer compression and more flexion injuries than the in-pool injuries. This is possibly related to the much softer bottoms in the natural environment and because many of these injuries happened to divers who launched themselves from the water bottom into the water while running on the beach or lake bottom. Estimated depth of water where the victim struck the bottom was derived from statements of witnesses. In 23(18.3%) of the 126 accidents occurring in a natural environment, the impact depth was 2 ft or less. In 107 (84.9%) of the accidents, the water was 4 ft deep or less.

Of the diving accidents reported by Gabrielsen[47] 67(13.8%) have been reconstructed by McElhaney et al.[11] by observing anthropometrically similar volunteers performing the same dives in deeper water. These include shallow water dives from the edge of the pool, springboard dives, and headfirst entry from a water slide. Dive kinematics were quantified using 200-frame-per-second film and a grid placed behind the diver (Figure 11.9). In this way, a lower bound for critical head impact velocity resulting in cervical injury has been developed. Based on these studies, in a clear dive, hydrodynamic drag generally does not start to slow the diver's in-water speed to values less than that at water entry until a significant portion of the diver's body is immersed. On the order of one half to three fourths of the body must be in the water when executing a clean dive before deceleration commences. Indeed, under the action of gravity, the diver's in-water head speed increases for the first few feet of penetration (Table 11.5).

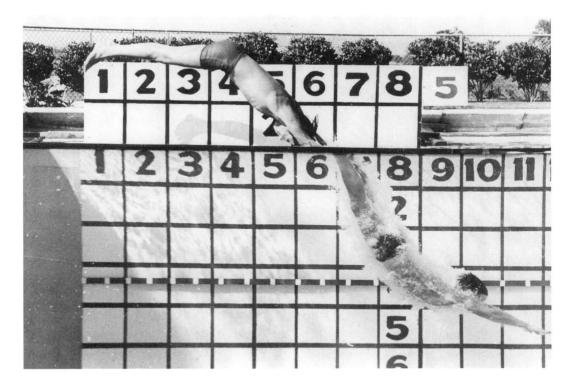

FIGURE 11.9 Diving accident reconstruction.

TABLE 11.5
Head Speeds for a 45 Degree Diving Entry

Depth (ft)	Head Speed (ft/s)
0.5	14.0
1.0	14.4
1.5	14.9
2.0	15.3
2.5	15.7
3.0	14.3
3.5	12.8
4.0	11.2
4.5	9.7
5.0	8.4
5.5	7.2
6.0	7.0
6.5	6.8

For dives from the edge of the pool, fall heights ranged from 116 cm (3.8 ft) to 219 cm (7.2 ft) (Figure 11.10). Estimated head impact speeds ranged from 3.11 m/s (10.2 ft/s) to 6.55 m/s (21.5 ft/s). Springboard and platform dives had a wide range of fall heights and water depths; however, impact velocities remained between 3.8 m/s (12.5 ft/s) and 8.1m/s (26.5 ft/s). Headfirst entry from a water

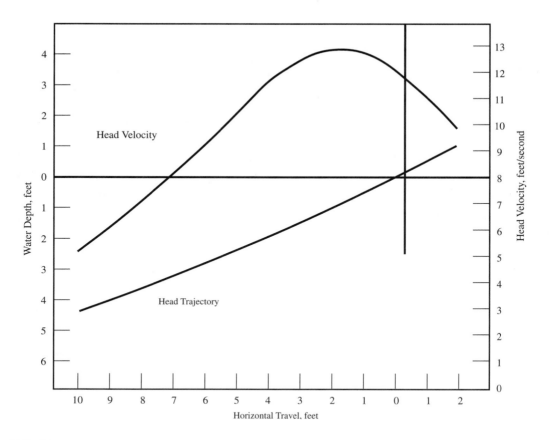

FIGURE 11.10: Head trajectory (lower curve, left axis) and velocity (upper curve, right axis) for a typical dive from the edge of a pool, showing the increase in head velocity following entry into the water.

slide has the potential for neck injury when, instead of skimming across the surface, the head and hands are lowered and a snap roll or tumble occurs. Head impact velocities for the snap roll mode range from 3.57 m/s (11.7 ft/s) to 4.94 m/s (16.2 ft/s).

It is clear from the number and severity of the accidents presented in this study that diving or headfirst sliding into shallow water is potentially dangerous and should be actively discouraged. The snap roll motion probably occurred in many of these accidents. Keeping the head and hands up and the back arched is critical in shallow water diving.

As noted, the neck injuries observed in diving are amazingly similar. There were only two head injuries, and no facial trauma was reported in the study. In the head-down impacts that probably occurred in the majority of these accidents, the forces were less than that required to cause head trauma but because of the body driving into the neck, catastrophic neck injuries occurred. In the head-up configuration, the face impacts the pool bottom with a glancing blow, the neck can extend, and the torso contacts the impact surface. Of course, this happens in the swimming pool environment. The lack, however, of serious, reported head and neck injuries connected with facial impacts indicates that the velocity range associated with diving is less than critical for this extension mode of injury, or perhaps that the neck's flexibility allows direct loading of the torso against the impact surface.

The results therefore indicate that flexion–compression injuries can occur with head impacts in a diving mode at velocities greater than 3.05 m/s (10 ft/s), where the head is suddenly stopped and the neck must stop the torso.

EXPERIMENTAL STUDIES

The neck injury literature includes numerous studies. Experimental investigations using whole cadavers have been invaluable in developing kinematic relationships as well as suggesting injury mechanisms. Additional experiments have used isolated spinal segments and cadaveric spines to examine specific factors influencing cervical injury. While these studies are extensive and diverse, a logical approach to cervical injury can be developed by considering the basic mechanical factors that influence injury.

SIMULATED INJURIES WITH CADAVERS

Flexion-Extension

Mertz and Patrick[48,49] have summarized data from forward and rearward sled decelerations of one human volunteer (Patrick) and four cadavers with weights added to the head at, above, or below the center of gravity of the head. These papers have come to define the corridors of the kinematic response and the recommended noninjurious tolerance values for head extension and flexion in dynamic and static loading situations. Posterior ligamentous injury occurred in the midcervical spine of a small cadaver with a measured peak occipital condylus moment of 33.2 N•m. This was scaled to 56.7 N•m to represent the 50th percentile male and was suggested as a threshold for ligamentous injury in extension. The largest deceleration applied to a cadaver produced a 189-N•m moment, with no evidence of injury detected by X-rays. This limit was suggested as the upper bound of ligamentous spine tolerance in flexion, despite the lack of injury.

Compression

Culver et al.[50] performed 11 superior–inferior head impacts of unembalmed cadavers using a padded impactor. Cadavers were placed in the supine position with the head and torso aligned with respect to the impactor. Posterior translation of the head was constrained, while anterior translation was not. No fractures were observed at peak head forces below 5.7 kN. Strain gauges were placed on the surface of three cervical vertebral bodies. Axial compression was applied anterior to the axis of the spine using either a fixed or pivoting head-end condition. Measurement of relative magnitudes of strain led the authors to conclude that increased padding on the crown in helmets did little to reduce neck injury and that increased constraint of the head in the padded impact surface increased the likelihood of neck injury.

Nusholtz et al.[51] performed impacts to the vertex of 12 unembalmed cadavers. A guided 56-kg instrumented impactor was used with impact velocities of 4.6 to 5.6 m/s. The impactor had a padded surface and incorporated a biaxial load cell. Extension–compression cervical injury occurred with the necks buckling in extension or flexion. Head impact loads ranged from 1.8 to 11.1 kN. Nusholtz et al.[27] also performed free fall drop tests using eight unembalmed cadavers with initial impact to the crown of the head. Drop heights that varied from 0.8 to 1.8 m produced extensive cervical and thoracic fractures and dislocations. Head impact forces varied from 3.2 to 10.8 kN in these tests. Nusholtz et al.[27] drew a variety of conclusions from these cadaver tests that still remain quite valid including

1. The initial orientation of the spine is a critical factor in influencing the dynamic response and injuries produced.
2. Descriptive motion of the head relative to the torso is not a good indicator of neck damage. For example, flexion damage can occur with extension motion and extension damage can occur with flexion motion.
3. Energy absorbing materials are effective methods for reducing peak impact force, but do not necessarily reduce the amount of energy transferred to the head, neck, and torso or the damage produced in a cadaver model.

Yoganandan et al.[52] (1986) conducted a study to evaluate the mechanism of spinal injuries with vertical impact. Sixteen fresh, intact, human male cadavers were suspended head down and dropped vertically from a height of 0.9 to 1.5 m. In 8 of the 16 specimens, the head was restrained to simulate the effect of muscle tone, producing preflexion of the cervical spine in its initial position. The head–neck complexes of the specimens were suitably oriented to achieve maximum axial loading of the cervical spine. Head–impact forces ranged from 3.0 to 7.1 kN in the unrestrained and from 9.8 to 14.7 kN in the restrained specimens. Cervical vertebral body damage was observed most commonly when the cadavers remained in contact with the impacting surface without substantial rotation or rebound. This caused the neck to be the major element in stopping the torso motion.

One important factor, not well controlled in all these compressive studies is the degree of head constraint. When the head is free to rotate on the condylus, bending of the neck occurs with minimum compression. When head rotation is constrained, bending of the neck is restricted and the system becomes much stiffer. The factors that influence head motion are the stiffness and conformability of the impacting surface and the cadaver head. Another factor that cannot be controlled in whole cadaver experiments is the extent to which failure progresses. A certain amount of kinetic energy is available and failures progress until this energy is dissipated. These factors, as well as lack of muscle action, make interpretation of injury mechanisms from whole cadaver tests difficult.

MECHANICAL FACTORS OF EXPERIMENTAL CERVICAL SPINAL INJURY

Mechanically, the spine may be thought of as a segmented structure composed of nonlinear viscoelastic elements and kinematic elements. The motion of the spine is coupled and the local deformations of the various elements produce large strains. Efforts to characterize this complex structure have included *in vivo* range of motion, cadaveric whole spines, motion segments, and isolated spinal ligament studies. Methodologies of evaluation have also been highly varied, and include quasi-static flexibility studies of isolated motion segments and static and dynamic testing of whole spines. Limitations in these methods are numerous and primarily include the method of reporting data. As an example, consider the flexion moment-angle relationship for a whole cervical spine in combined bending. Clearly the use of a single value to describe the stiffness/flexibility of this structure is inadequate. Thus, to provide meaningful data it is necessary that studies include a detailed description of testing and the method of derivation.

These limitations notwithstanding, significant contributions to understanding spinal structural properties have been made. These are best discussed by considering the spine as a beam–column and examining the mechanical factors affecting this system and its viscoelastic effects. Mechanical factors to be addressed include loading rate, musculature effects, load position, head motion, buckling, initial position, and end condition (or the degree of head constraint).

Loading Rate

The cervical spine and its constituents exhibit rate-dependent, viscoelastic effects when loaded. For this reason, the results of a study by McElhaney et al.,[26] where compression testing of whole cervical spines was performed, are discussed in some detail. This study demonstrates the effects of viscoelasticity on the cervical spine. Load relaxation, the decrease in load with constant deformation, is indicative of the prominence of viscoelastic effects. Differences in load that would be observed between high rates and quasi-static tests are on the order of 70%. Load relaxation is initially extremely rapid; thereafter, load decays at a much slower rate. This type of rate behavior renders a standard lumped parameter viscoelastic model with a single dominant long-term time constant a poor predictor of neck behavior. Instead, a generalized Maxwell–Weichert model must be used because it incorporates an ensemble of relaxation time constants.

In addition to having a significant component of viscoelasticity, the spine also demonstrates a second component of time dependence, preconditioning. Following large periods (hours) of inactivity, additional fluid is absorbed by the soft tissues of the spine, placing it in a stiffened state, the fully reequilibrated state. Following activity the additional fluid is extruded from the structure and the stiffness of the structure decreases. Eventually, a steady state is reached in which subsequent activity does not produce a change in stiffness. This is the mechanically stabilized or preconditioned state. By defining the cyclic modulus as the peak load over the peak deflection during sinusoidal loading, the cyclic modulus of the mechanically stabilized state ranged from 45 to 55% of the fully reequilibrated state. Given that most individuals are continually active, all structural testing should be performed in the mechanically stabilized state.

Given the viscoelastic nature of the constituents of the cervical spine, it is not surprising that its structural and failure properties are sensitive to loading rate. An increase in loading velocity has been reported to increase the stiffness, failure load, and energy at failure for a variety of spinal tissues. For example, the intervertebral disk exhibits increased stiffness with rate of loading in compression.[53] Bone exhibits increased stiffness and ultimate load with increased compression rate.[54,55] Similar behavior has been associated with the spinal ligaments in tension.[56] Chang et al.[57] reported increased stiffness of the cervical spine with increased rate of loading. Indeed, McElhaney et al.[26] reported that varying the loading rate by a factor of 500 resulted in a change in spinal stiffness from 1285 to 2250 N/cm for a single specimen. A significant positive correlation between failure load and loading rate for the cervical spine in nearly pure compressive loading has been reported by Pintar et al.[58] By using a linear regression model with loading rates varying from 2 mm/s to 8 m/s, forces to failure ranged from 2.2 kN at 2 mm/s to 5.4 kN at 8 m/s.

Load Position and Combined Loading

Loading of the cervical spine, either as a result of head inertia or head impact, results in a state of combined loading in which forces and bending moments act simultaneously. The three kinds of forces acting on the spine (compression–tension, lateral shear, and anteroposterior shear) can be replaced by a single vector resultant. Further, that resultant can be located in space such that the moments of the resultant force are equal to the moments imposed by the three components of force and the three applied moments (torsion, lateral bending, and flexion–extension). For many loading conditions, the significant components of the resultant force are located in the sagittal plane. Defining the eccentricity as the perpendicular distance from the sagittal plane resultant force to the spine, yields a quantity that can explain the mechanism of injury of the cervical spine.

Based on a review of other published works, Myers and Winkelstein[23] reported that this has been particularly well demonstrated for neck loading resulting in combined bending and axial compression of the cervical spine. Specifically, increasing eccentricity of the resultant force from posterior to anterior changes the injury mechanism from posterior element failure to vertebral body compression fractures, burst fractures, and wedge compression fractures; and, when it is located most anteriorly, to facet dislocations (Figure 11.11).

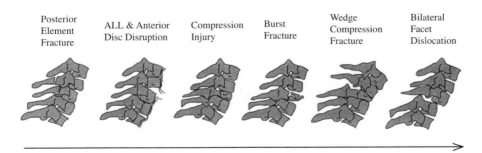

| Posterior Element Fracture | ALL & Anterior Disc Disruption | Compression Injury | Burst Fracture | Wedge Compression Fracture | Bilateral Facet Dislocation |

Increasing Anterior Eccentricity

FIGURE 11.11 Schematic drawings of injuries illustrate the influence of increasing eccentricity, from posterior to anterior, of compressive force on cervical spinal injury.

McElhaney et al.[26] subjected preflexed cervical spines to compressive displacements and produced burst fractures. These fractures were produced with a slight anterior eccentricity of load; yet no quantitative data were provided. McElhaney et al.[26] also reported that moving the load vector 1.0 cm or more posterior to the vertebral body resulted in posterior element fractures; and tears of the anterior longitudinal ligament and disk anteriorly, which are due to the tensile stresses associated with the extension moment. Therefore, these posterior element fractures may be considered compression–extension injuries with a resultant force located behind the vertebral bodies. Bates-Carter et al.[59] produced burst fractures in isolated lower cervical spine specimens, noting that burst fractures were reliably produced when the spine was tested in a preflexed position and axially impacted with the line of force anterior to the center of the vertebral body. These injuries resulted from compressive loads with eccentricities less than 1.0 cm anterior to the midpoint of the vertebral bodies. Similar observations were made by Pintar et al.[30] using their head–neck impact model. McElhaney et al.[26] reported that eccentricities of the resultant force of approximately 1.0 cm anterior to those that produced burst fractures produce wedge compression fractures. With further increases in the eccentricity of the resultant load, bilateral facet dislocations are produced. While not reporting an average value of eccentricity, Myers et al.[44] showed that the eccentricity of the resultant force was in excess of 6.0 cm anterior to the vertebral body at the time of injury. Flexion bending moments were suggested as the dominant form of loading resulting in bilateral facet dislocations.

Buckling and Buckled Deformation

Injuries observed in real-world head impacts are often multiple and noncontiguous, and the result of various mechanisms at different levels within the spine.[60,61] Concomitant flexion and extension injuries have been both observed in clinical studies and produced in experimental studies.[28,45,61,62] The cervical spine may be considered as a slender beam column with a fixed base (the torso end) and pinned apex (the head end). Once the critical load is reached, this structure can snap-through buckle with a rapid transition from a predominantly compressive mode of deformation to a predominantly bending mode of deformation. Torg[5] and Torg et al.[63,64] wrote extensively that buckling of the cervical spine causes neck injury. While it has been demonstrated that buckling is a structural failure, it is not a material failure (a neck injury). Because the buckle occurs prior to injury,[28,44,45] the cervical spine shows postbuckling stability and can undergo buckling without injury.

While buckling is not injury, the postbuckled deformation pattern does explain the mechanism of injuries that occur after buckling. The deformation pattern of the spine following the buckle is a first-mode buckle for a fixed-pinned column (Figure 11.12). The buckled deformation of the spine exhibits regions of extension in the upper cervical spine and flexion in the lower cervical spine. As a result, the neck load vector passes behind the upper cervical spine causing upper cervical compression–extension, and in front of the lower cervical spine causing lower cervical compression–flexion. Thus, with continued increases in load, the post–buckled spine fails, and the failures may be either compression–extension or compression–flexion. Therefore, while buckling has never been demonstrated experimentally to cause material failure in the neck, it plays a role in determining which types of injuries are produced. It also provides an additional mechanistic explanation for the absence of a relationship between head motion and compression-bending neck injury.

End Condition

The internal loads of the cervical spine are governed by the imposed end conditions of the head–neck–torso system. The approximation of the torso as a fixed end condition has been used by several investigators in cadaver tests and typically results in the production of realistic cervical injuries.[28–30,44,45,65,66] The rationale for this approximation is that the large rotary inertia of the torso precludes significant torso rotations in the short time in which neck injuries occur. While this

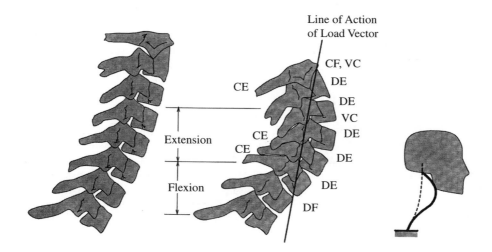

FIGURE 11.12 Illustration of initial configuration and deformation of the first buckling mode for the cervical spine, modeled by a fixed-pinned column, with regions of extension in the upper cervical spine and flexion in the lower cervical spine.

appears reasonable for neck injuries due to head impact, it is likely less valid for the longer duration dynamic events like noncontact frontal decelerations. The head geometry, mass, and interaction with a contact surface confound the simple definition of the upper cervical end condition; and as a result, investigators have imposed a variety of different end conditions on the head in an effort to better understand the importance of this factor on neck injury.

Mechanical analysis based on the effective mass of the torso and the energy absorption of the neck reveals that the cervical spine is capable of managing impacts equivalent to vertical drop of 0.50 m when the neck is called on to stop the torso.[11] Unfortunately, most impact situations have considerably larger impact energies. Put in its simplest terms, because of the large mass of the torso, the head and neck must either escape from the path of the moving torso or be at risk for injury. Therefore, restriction of the motion of the head in the escape direction may increase the risk for neck injury.

Impact Surface Stiffness and Padding Characteristics

Because of the obvious benefits in reduction of head injury risk and the high frequency of head injuries as compared with neck injuries, padding is often added to a potential impact surface. However, the addition of compliant pads to the impact surface may increase the risk of injury to the cervical spine. The mechanism by which this increase in risk occurs may be more involved than the end condition–head constraint mechanism (so-called "pocketing"). In impacts with a compliant surface, the head pockets into the pad, and its motion parallel to the impact surface is opposed by both pressure and surface friction effects. In other words, the deformed padding applies forces to the head that oppose the escape velocity of the head.

Padding, by virtue of a change in stiffness and not by pocketing, also delays the escape of the head from the impact surface. Specifically, by lowering the stiffness, the magnitude of the head force is diminished and the contact time is increased. As a result, the motion of the head in the escape direction, as a result of impact surface forces in the escape direction, is delayed and diminished. Nightingale et al.[34] have shown that for impacts near the vertex of the head there is a significant increase in the frequency and severity of neck injuries sustained in padded impacts when compared with rigid impacts. This finding is particularly clear in the cases where the head is impacted posteriorly. The velocity in the escape direction flexes the head, allowing the head and neck to escape out of the way of the following torso. However, in padded impacts the deformed padding applies forces directed posteriorly and increases the time the head spends in the contact surface. As a result, the neck sees a significantly larger torso impulse and suffers injuries. It should be recognized that the materials used in these experiments were considerably more compliant than those used currently in automotive and other safety environments. However, it should also be apparent that the addition of surface padding cannot be considered as a method of protecting the neck from injury.

Studies have identified impact surface friction as a contributor to neck injury risk in compressive impacts. Indeed, increases in the coefficient of friction between the head and the impact surface greater than or equal to 0.5 were found to constrain the head translation[67] prohibiting motion in the escape direction. Increases in the coefficient of friction were reported to increase both the neck forces and occiput-C-1 moments. The mechanism for increased risk for neck injury is due to frictional forces constraining the head and preventing escape from the following torso. Moreover, in a parametric analysis, including pad thickness and surface friction, increases in the coefficient of friction had the most profound effect on increasing neck forces and moments.[68] This study further reported that for increases in pad thickness, head forces were decreased with no increase in neck injury risk. In that regard, the historically cited pocketing mechanism relates more to friction than to the depth of the padding.

Impact Attitude and Head Inertia

While increased constraint and increased contact time may increase neck injury risk, they are by no means requisite for neck injury. The effects of head inertia and the impact surface attitude (or equivalently, the direction of the velocity of the body relative to the impact surface) are important determinants of neck injury risk. Head inertial loads alone have been shown by Nightingale et al.[34,45] to constrain cervical spine motion and produce neck injury in the absence of any constraints imposed by the impact surface. The attitude of the impact surface has a profound effect on the risk for neck injury. Attitudes in which the cervical spine is oriented more closely to perpendicular to the impact surface place the neck at greater risk for injury than those in which the orientation of the spine is less perpendicular to the impact surface.[27,28,45,51] Recognizing that the neutrally positioned cervical spine has a flexion rotation of approximately 25 degrees anterior, in a vertex impact, the neck-loading vector has only a small component of force in the direction required to accelerate the head and neck out of the path of the following torso. In contrast, for impacts posterior to the head vertex, the head has a component of velocity in the anterior direction that is immediately increased by the neck-loading vector. As a result, the head and neck are more likely to escape the torso loading in impacts posterior to the crown of the head. If the impact surface attitude is sufficiently far enough forward that the face hits the contact surface, the probability of neck injury is again decreased through a similar extension mechanism. This observation is supported by an analysis of shallow water diving accidents reported by McElhaney et al.[11] in which divers suffering facial injuries did not suffer neck injuries, and divers with neck injuries did not suffer facial injuries.

TOLERANCE OF THE CERVICAL SPINE

Characterization of the tolerance of the human cervical spine to injury remains a challenge to biomechanical engineering. Tolerance, in addition to being a function of the loading environment, is related to a variety of host-related factors. These include, but are not limited to, the bone mineral content of the vertebra, the presence of degeneration, the degree of muscular stimulation at the time of impact, and the variance associated with the geometric differences within the population. In addition, males and females constitute different populations in terms of cervical spine tolerance. A study by Nightingale et al.[31] showed a significant difference between the failure loads of the male and female spine. Compressive failure loads averaged 1.06 kN for females and 2.24 kN for males. An additional limitation on tolerance research is the lack of availability of cadaveric tissue for the study of injury. This lack of tissue severely restricts the size of most studies and is, perhaps, the greatest limitation on advancing our understanding of injury biomechanics. Despite all these limitations, a great deal has been learned about the tolerance of the neck to injury. The following is a summary of a number of studies reporting data relevant to the question of human cervical spine tolerance.

COMPRESSION

A large number of studies have reported compressive load to failure. While it is readily accepted that this parameter alone is a poor predictor of the risk for neck injury, it still remains a readily measurable and useful biomechanical parameter. Understanding and interpreting these data can reduce the observed scatter and provide some insight into compressive cervical tolerance.

Differences in axial load to failure have been shown to depend on the injury produced and, therefore, on the degree of constraint imposed by the contact surface. From a tolerance standpoint, these injuries should be evaluated separately. As an example, cadaver experiments by Maiman et al.,[69] Myers et al.,[44] and Pintar et al.,[70] show that compression–flexion and compression–extension injuries occur with smaller axial loads than pure compressive injuries do. In contrast, the compressive loads associated with pure compression injuries are a reasonable estimate of cervical compressive tolerance.

Further reduction in the scatter of compressive data may be gained by considering the effects of rate on axial load to failure. This concerns two primary effects. First, increasing rates of loading from quasi-static to dynamic (from 0 to 5 or 10 Hz, loading duration of 200 ms) results in increases in measured axial load of as much as 50% due to viscous effects. Second, increasing loading rate to impact velocities (loading durations of approximately 20 ms or less) includes inertial effects of the head. Impactor load data must then be interpreted with the realization that neck loading depends heavily on the inertial characteristics and accelerations of the head. The force measured at the point of head contact is considerably larger than the force transmitted to the neck because the neck force is reduced by the product of head mass and the head acceleration. Accordingly, data must be interpreted with the realization that neck loading is greatly reduced and depends on the inertial characteristics and accelerations of the head and impactor. This effect is evident in the studies that have simultaneously measured the head impact load and the neck load. Yoganandan et al.[50] reported peak head loads and orientations; it is important to use data from studies that employ similar experimental setups. Motion segment studies are limited because the specimens are too short to exhibit buckling behavior. Studies of isolated spines are also limited because they do not include the important dynamic effects of the intact head. In the studies that use whole heads and cervical spines, the most confounding problem leading to the scatter in tolerance data is the use of force data from the head or impactor. If analysis is limited to the studies that (1) are dynamic, (2) include the head mass, (3) do not constrain the motion of the head, and (4) include instrumentation to measure the loads in the cervical spine, the scatter in the data is sufficiently reduced to allow the formulation of a tolerance for predominantly compressive loading. The studies that meet these criteria are Nightingale et al.,[31] Pintar et al.[66,70] and Yoganandan et al.[71,72] A synthesis of these data is presented in Nightingale et al.[31] and is briefly summarized in the next paragraph.

The mean failure loads reported in the Pintar and Yoganandan studies are higher than the values reported by Nightingale et al.[31] However, this is due to the fact that the former studies used preflexed spines while the latter used curved, neutrally positioned spines. Because the initial curvature of the cervical spine in the injury environment is unknown, the results of the two studies were combined to formulate a tolerance for males and females. Averaging the means of the two studies resulted in the following tolerance values: 1.68 kN for females, and 3.03 kN for males. The tolerance values were scaled to account for the age of the cadaver specimens and the authors suggest a cervical spine tolerance for the young human male in the range of 3.64 to 3.94 kN. The tolerance will likely be lower for a neutrally positioned spine and higher for a straightened spine; however, it is a representation of the mean resultant force required for a catastrophic cervical spine injury in any given impact situation.

SUMMARY

Cervical injury mechanisms involve a wide range of loading modes with various combinations of load and concurrent bending moment. Using the classical concepts of excessive head motion as a cause of neck injury frequently leads to paradoxical and incorrect observations concerning the injury. In contrast, when the neck is viewed as a mechanical structure, whose injury is a consequence of the vibrations of a segmented beam column bounded by two large masses, these paradoxical observations can be readily explained. That is, by considering the effects of buckling and examining the forces and moments that act locally on the spine at the time of injury, each injury may be uniquely classified. Understanding human cervical tolerance has developed significantly, and new injury criteria are actively being discussed at the time of this publication.

Much work remains to be done. Improvements in computational models of neck dynamics have been dramatic and remain promising. These models, however, remain only as good as the data on which they are developed. The concepts of pocketing and the constraints imposed by the impact surface have been refined and have identified surface friction as an important source of constraints that can increase injury risk. These same studies also show that conventional materials cannot provide the benefits possible, and future research to develop injury prevention strategies that capitalize on these results will be required. Understanding the effects of the spinal musculature, tensile neck injuries, and the unique features of the pediatric spine also remain as goals for the next decade.

In shallow water diving, catastrophic cervical injuries generally occur in the rare circumstances when the head is impacted and the cervical spine is trapped between the slowed or stopped head and the moving torso. To accomplish this the head force vector must be aligned with a stiff axis of the neck and torso.

ACKNOWLEDGMENTS

This work was supported by the Department of Health and Human Services, Center of Disease Control Grant R49/CCR402396-12, and the Virginia Flowers Baker Chair at Duke University.

REFERENCES

1. National Spinal Cord Injury Statistical Center (NSCISC), Spinal Cord Injury: Facts and Figures at a Glance, University of Alabama at Birmingham, April 1999, www.spinalcord.uab.edu.
2. Berkowitz, M., O'Leary, P. K., Kruse, D. L., and Harvey, C., *Spinal Cord Injury: An Analysis of Medical and Social Costs*, Demos Medical Publ. New York, NY, 1998.
3. Allen, D. G., Reid, D. C., and Saboe, L., 1988.
4. Shield, L. K., Fox, B., and Stauffer, E. S., Cervical cord injury in sports, *Physician Sports Med.*, 6, 321, 1978.
5. Torg, J. S., Mechanisms and pathomechanics of athletic injuries to the cervical spine, in *Athletic Injuries to the Head, Neck and Face*, Lea & Febiger, Philadelphia, 1982, chap. 11.
6. Torg, J. S. 1979.
7. Torg, J. S. 1979.
8. Torg, J. S. 1985.
9. Kewalramani, and Taylor, 1975.
10. Albrand, O. W. and Walter, J., Underwater deceleration curves in relation to injuries from diving, *Surgical Neurol*, 4, 461, 1975.
11. McElhaney, J. H., Snyder, R. G., States, J. D., and Gabrielsen, M. A., Biomechanical Analysis of Swimming Pool Injuries, SAE Paper 790137, 1979, 47.
12. Gabrielsen, M. A. and McElhaney, J. H., The Effect of Water Slide Configuration on the Velocity and Depth of Penetration, CPSC Report No. 644, February 1974.
13. Reid, D. C. and Saboe, L. Spine fractures in winter sports, *Sports Med.*, 7(6), 393, 1989.

14. White, A. A., III and Panjabi, M. M., *Clinical Biomechanics of the Spine*, 2nd ed., Lippincott, Philadelphia, 1990.
15. Babcock, J. L., Cervical spine injuries: diagnosis and classification, *Arch. Surg.*, 111, 646, 1976.
16. Melvin, J. W., Mohan, D., and Stalnaker, R. L., Occupant injury mechanisms and impact tolerance, *Transp., Res., Rec.* (Transportation Research Board), 586, 11, 1976.
17. Moffatt, C. A., Advani, S. H., and Lin, C.J., Analytical End Experimental Investigations of Human Spine Flexure, American Society of Mechanical Engineers Paper No. 71-WA/BHF-7, 1971.
18. Portnoy, H. D., McElhaney, J. H., Melvin, J. W., and Croissant, P. D., Mechanism of cervical spine injury in auto accidents, Proc. 15th Annual Conf. American Association for Automotive Medicine, 1972, 58.
19. Allen, 1982.
20. White, A. A., III and Panjabi, M. M., 1978.
21. Dolen, K. D., Cervical spine injuries below the axis, *Rad. Clin. No. Am.* 15(2), 247, 1977.
22. Harris, 1986.
23. Myers, B. S., and Winkelstein, B. A., Epidemiology, classification, mechanism, and tolerance of human cervical spine injuries, *Crit. Rev. Biomed. Eng.*, 23(5–6), 307, 1995.
24. Yoganandan, N. 1989.
25. Stedman, 1982.
26. McElhaney, J. H., Paver, J. G., McCrackin, H. J., and Maxwell, G. M., Cervical spine compression responses, Proc. 27th Stapp Car Crash Conf., SAE Paper 831615, 1983, 163.
27. Nusholtz, G. S., Huelke, D. F., Lux, P., Alem, N. M., and Montalvo, F., Cervical spine injury mechanisms, Proc. 27th Stapp Car Crash Conf., SAE Paper 831616, 1983, 179.
28. Nightingale, R. W., McElhaney, J. H., Richardson, W. J., Best, T. M., and Myers, B. S., Experimental cervical spine injury: relating head motion, injury classification, and injury mechanism, *J. Bone Joint Surg.*, 78-A(3), 412, 1996.
29. Yoganandan, N., Sances, A., Jr., and Pintar, F., Biomechanical evaluation of the axial compressive responses of the human cadaveric and manikin necks, *J. Biomech. Eng.*, 111, 250, 1989.
30. Pintar, F. A., Yoganandan, N., Voo, L., Cusick, J. F., Maiman, D. J., and Sances, A., Jr., Dynamic characteristics of the human cervical spine, Proc. 39th Stapp Car Crash Conf., SAE Paper 952722, 1995, 195.
31. Nightingale, R. W., McElhaney, J. H., Camacho, D. L., Winkelstein, B. A., and Myers, B. S., The dynamic responses of the cervical spine: the role of buckling, end conditions, and tolerance in compressive impacts, Proc. 41st Stapp Car Crash Conf., SAE Paper 973344, 1997, 451.
32. Jefferson, 1920.
33. Myers, B. S., and Nightingalel, R. W., Basilar skull fracture resulting from compressive neck loading, AGARD Specialist Meet. Impact Head Injury, Mescalero, NM, November 1997, 3-1–3-10.
34. Nightingale, R. W., Richardson, W. J., and Myers, B. S., The effects of padded surfaces on the risk for cervical spine injury, *Spine*, 22(10), 2380, 1997.
35. Braakman, R. and Penning, L., Causes of spinal lesions, in *Injuries of the Cervical Spine*, Exerpta Medica, Amsterdam, 53, 1971.
36. Crowell, R. R., Coffee, M. S., Edwards, W. T., and White, A. A., III, Proc. Cervical Spine Research Society, 1987.
37. Braakman, R. and Vinken, P. J., Unilateral facet interlocking in the lower cervical spine, *J. Bone Joint Surg.*, 49B(2), 249, 1967.
38. Huelke, D. F., Moffett, E. A., Mendelshon, R. A., and Melvin, J. W., Cervical fractures and fracture dislocations: an overview, SAE Paper 790131, 1979, 462.
39. Gosch, 1972.
40. Roaf, R., A study of the mechanics of spinal injury, *J. Bone Joint Surg.*, 42B, 810, 1960.
41. Rogers, 1957.
42. Bauze, R. J., and Ardran, G. M., Experimental production of forward dislocation of the human cervical spine, *J. Bone Joint Surg.*, 60B, 239, 1978.
43. Myers, B. S. 1991.
44. Myers, B. S., McElhaney, J. H., Richardson, W. J., Nightingale, R. W., and Doherty, B. J., The influence of end condition on human cervical spine injury mechanisms, Proc. 35th Stapp Car Crash Conf., SAE Paper 912915, 1991, 391.

45. Nightingale, R. W., McElhaney, J. H., Richardson, W. J., and Myers, B. S., Dynamic responses of the head and cervical spine to axial impact loading, *J. Biomech*, 29(3), 307, 1996.
46. Nahm, A. and Melvin, *J., Accidental Injury, Biomechanics and Prevention,* Springer-Verlag, Berlin, 1990.
47. Gabrielsen, M. A., *Diving Injuries: The Etiology of 486 Case Studies with Recommendations for Needed Action*, NOVA University Press, Ft. Lauderdale, FL, 1990.
48. Mertz, H. J. and Patrick, L. M., 1967.
49. Mertz, H. J., and Patrick, L. M., Strength and response of the human neck, Proc 15th Stapp Car Crash Conf., SAE Paper 710855, 1971, 1971, 207.
50. Culver, C. C., Bender, M., and Melvin, J. W. Mechanisms, tolerances, and responses obtained under dynamic superior-inferior head impact, UM-HSRI-78-21, 1978.
51. Nushotz, G. S. 1981.
52. Yoganandan, N., Sances, A., Jr., Maiman, D. J., Myklebust, J. B., Pech, P., and Larson, S. J., Experimental spinal injuries with vertical impact, *Spine*, 11(9), 855, 1986.
53. Casper, R. A., The Viscoelastic Behavior of the Human Intervertebral Disc, Ph.D. dissertation, Duke University, Durham, NC, 1980.
54. Kazarian, L. and Graves, 1977.
55. Kaplan, F. S., Hayes, W. C., Keaveny, T. M., Boskey, A., Einhorn, T. A., and Iannotti, J. P., Form and function of bone, *Orthopaedic Basic Science*, American Academy of Orthopaedic Surgeons, 1994.
56. Yoganandan, N., Pintar, F., Butler, J., Reinartz, J., Sances, A., Jr., and Larson, S. J., Dynamic response of human cervical spine ligaments, *Spine*, 14(10), 1102, 1989.
57. Chang, 1992.
58. Pintar, F. A. 1996.
59. Bates-Carter, 1995.
60. Bohlman, 1973.
61. Levine, A. M., and Edwards, C. C., Fractures of the atlas, *J. Bone Joint Surg.*, 73(5), 680, 1991.
62. Shear, 1988.
63. Torg, J. S. 1990.
64. Torg, J. S. 1993.
65. Pintar, F. A., Yoganandan, N., Sances, A., Jr., Reinartz, J., Larson, S. J., and Harris, G., Kinematic and anatomical analysis of the human cervical spinal column under axial loading, Proc. 33rd Stapp Car Crash Conf., SAE Paper 892436, 1989, 987.
66. Pintar, F. A. 1990.
67. Camacho, 1999.
68. Camacho, in preparation.
69. Maiman, D. J., Sances, A., Myklebust, J. B., Larson, S. J., Houterman, C., Chilbert, M., and El-Ghatit, A. Z., Compression injuries of the cervical spine; a biomechanical analysis. *Neurosurgery*, 13(3), 254, 1983.
70. Pintar, F. A. 1995.
71. Yoganandan, N., Pintar, F. A., Sances, A., Jr., Reinartz, J., and Larson, S. J., Strength and kinematic response of dynamic cervical spine injuries, *Spine*, 16(10), S511, 1991.
72. Yoganandan, N. 1990.
73. Huelke, D. F., Mendelsohn, R. A., States, J. D., and Melvin, J. W. Cervical fractures and fracture dislocations sustained without head impact, in Human Neck, Anatomy, Injury Mechanisms and Biomechanics, SAE Special Paper 790132, 1979, S.P. 438.
74. Kazarian, L., Classification of simple spinal injuries, in *Impact Injury of the Head and Spine*, Ewing, C. L., Thomas, D. J., Sances, A., and Larson, S. J., eds., Charles C. Thomas, Springfield, IL, 1983, 72.
75. McElhaney, J. H., Doherty, B. J., Paver, J. G., Myers, B. S., and Gray, L., Combined bending and axial loading responses of the human cervical spine, Proc. 32nd Stapp Car Crash Conf., SAE Paper 881709, 1988, 21.
76. McElhaney, J. H., Roberts, V. L., Paver, J. G., and Maxwell, G. M., Etiology of trauma to the cervical spine, in *Impact Injury of the Head and Spine*, Ewing, C. L., Thomas, D. L., Sances, A., Jr., and Larson, S. J., Eds., Charles C Thomas, Springfield, IL, 1983.
77. McElhaney, J. H., Doherty, B. J., Paver, J. G., Myers, B. S., and Gray, L., Flexion, extension and lateral bending responses of the cervical spine, 67th Proc. NATO-AGARD Conf. Neck Injuries Advanced Military Aircraft Environments, Munich; and Proc. 2nd Int. Symp. Prevention of Head and Neck Injuries in Sports, Toronto, 1989.

78. Schneider, R. C., *Head and Neck Injuries in Football*, Williams & Wilkins, Baltimore, 1973.
79. Torg, J. S., ed., *Athletic Injuries to the Head, Neck and Face*, Philadelphia, Lea & Febiger, 1982.
80. Torg, J. S. and Pavlov, H., Axial load teardrop fracture, in *Athletic Injuries to the Head, Neck and Face*, 2nd ed., Lea & Febiger, Philadelphia, 1991.
81. Torg, J. S., Sennett, B., and Vegso, J. J., Spinal injury at the level of the third and fourth cervical vertebrae resulting from the axial loading mechanism: an analysis and classification, *Clin Sports Med.*, 6(1), 159, 1987.
82. Winkelstein, B. A., Nightingale, R. W., Richardson, W. J., and Myers, B. S., A biomechanical investigation of the cervical facet capsule and its role in whiplash injury, *Spine*, in review.

12 Recommendations for Reducing the Number of Pool Diving Injuries

WHAT THE DATA REVEALED

It was imperative for the authors and the Editorial Board to examine carefully the data concerning swimming pool injuries presented in Chapters 4 to 8 before any recommendations were made for changes in pool design or operation. After careful analysis of the data, certain undeniable facts were arrived at relative to how, where, and to whom these 440 catastrophic injuries occurred. The most essential findings from the review of the data and the authors' experience follow.

1. Of the 440 pool diving injuries recorded in this book, 365(83.0%) occurred in these three locations:

   - residential pools—228(51.8%)
   - motel/hotel pools—72(16.4%)
   - apartment/condominium pools—65(14.8%)

2. Less than 2% of the 365 pools listed in 1. had lifeguards to supervise the users of the pool.
3. Of the 440 pool cases, 92(20.9%) of the victims were injured when diving from springboards or jumpboards.
4. As to the injuries resulting from dives off springboards/jumpboards, all the victims struck the upslope of the pool bottom, the transition of the bottom from the deepest point to the shallow portion of the pool (see Appendix B). These pools had either a spoon-shaped or a hopper-bottom configuration (see Figures 12.1 and 12.2).
5. The water depth of the pool where 337(76.6%) of the victims struck the bottom was 4 ft deep or less, with 292(66.4%) striking the bottom at 3 ft 6 in. or less.

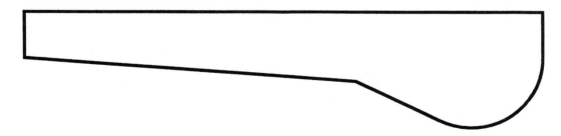

FIGURE 12.1 Diving envelope for spoon-shaped pools.

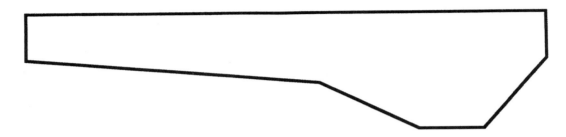

FIGURE 12.2 Diving envelope for hopper-bottom pools.

6. With respect to the injuries that occurred in 105 aboveground pools, 67(63.8%) were dives from a deck attached to the rim of the pool or from the top of a ladder extending into the pool.

7. In 5 of the 105 aboveground pool injuries, the center of the pool bottom was dug out creating a depth of approximately 5 ft to 5 ft 6 in. deep. This configuration is known as a variable bottom depth. Some people interpreted this to mean they could dive into the pool.

8. With respect to the injuries resulting from dives off starting blocks that were 30 in. above the water surface, all occurred in water depths that were 4 ft or less, with most at 3 ft 6 in.

9. In 215(48.9%) of the pools, there were no rules posted anywhere around the pool that would identify the proper use of the facilities to patrons, which was a disturbing fact.

10. Signs prohibiting diving from any place in the pool were present in only 43(9.8%) of the 440 accident sites.

11. With respect to the consumption of any form of alcoholic beverages, 179(40.7%) of the victims, by their own admission, had a drink or two during a 6-h period prior to sustaining his injury. Most claimed it was beer.

12. Only seven (1.6%) of the victims admitted to having used any drugs during a similar period.

13. As was expected, most of the victims (327, 74.3%) were rescued and removed from the pool by friends, who invariably failed to use a spineboard to remove the diver from the water. Only a few of the pools had any spineboard in the pool area.

14. The predominate injury levels to the spine were at the C-5, C-5, 6, and C-6 vertebrae.

15. In 137(31.1%) of the injuries, the level of lighting of the pool was below acceptable standards, which was disturbing to learn.

16. Only a few of the victims had ever received any instruction in diving from a qualified instructor.

17. The mean age of the male victims was 23.8; and that of the female, 20.9.

18. Interviews with the victims revealed the following:

   - They never thought that they could break their neck by diving where they did.
   - No one told them verbally not to dive.
   - They claimed that if they had seen a sign prohibiting diving they would not have done so.
   - A surprising number indicated that their hands struck the bottom of the pool first and slipped.
   - The accident happened on the victim's first visit to the pool and most, on the first dive they made into the pool.

19. The profiles of the victims and of the pools involved in the accidents are contained in Appendix A.
20. Finally, it was a surprise to find that many of the victims had only a bump on the head and none had abrasions or lacerations. From this it can be concluded that it does not take much force on the head to cause damage to the spine (see Chapter 10).

Many of the defects and pool omissions that were found have been corrected in the last 10 years, because pool owners and operators have become more aware of what is safe practice in the design and management of pools.

MAJOR POOL DESIGN CHANGES NEEDED FOR REDUCING POOL DIVING ACCIDENTS

The authors and members of the Editorial Board have given much thought to the need to improve both the design of swimming pools and their manner of operation. Some of the recommendations we have made may appear to be extreme; nevertheless, some drastic measures are required if pools are to be made and operated in a much safer manner. What we have concluded to be the essential changes that must be made are discussed next.

SPECIFICATIONS OF THE DIVING WELL

The construction of vinyl-liner, hopper-bottom and spoon-shaped pools as now designed (see Figures 12.1 and 12.2) should be discontinued. All those who design and construct pools with diving equipment (either springboards or jumpboards) are urged to follow the specifications set forth in Figure 12.3. Those who have diving equipment installed in pools that do not meet these specifications should be instructed to remove the boards, or at a minimum restrict their use to children under the age of 12. If these recommendations are implemented, it would practically ensure the elimination of all injuries resulting from dives from springboards/jumpboards.

POOL BOTTOM MARKINGS

All pools should have markings on the bottom to enable anyone contemplating a dive to better visualize the bottom and to assist the diver to more accurately ascertain the depth of the water. See Figure 12.4 for suggested markings for hopper-bottom pools and Figures 12.5 and 12.6 for above-ground pools.

STARTING BLOCKS

Starting blocks for competitive swimming must be located at the deep end of the pool where the water is at least 6 ft deep. If the recommended depth cannot be achieved, blocks should be removed and swimming races should be started from the deck of the pool. This would ensure the elimination of all injuries occurring as a consequence of dives off starting blocks.

POOL WATER SLIDES

All water slides should be placed in the deep end of pools where water is at least 8 ft deep. No slides should be located in the shallow end of the pool. The height of slides should be limited to 8 ft and use limited to the sitting position only. If small slides (4 to 6 ft in height) are used for children, they may be placed in water 4 ft deep and restricted to children in sitting positions only. Ladders, top transition "seat," and handrails should be slip resistant.

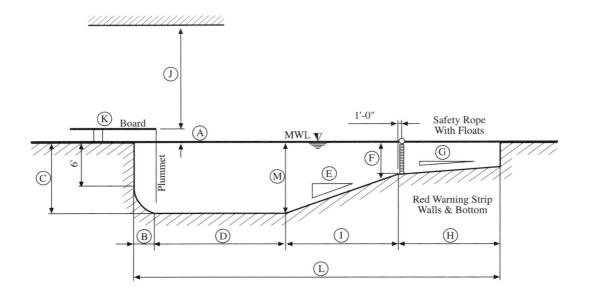

Dimension	Measurements
A. Height of above water	20 inches
B. Board overhang	3 feet
C. Depth of water at plummet	10 feet
D. Distance from plummet to upslope	16 feet
E. Inclination of upslope of bottom	1:3
F. Depth of water at breakpoint	4 feet
G. Slope of bottom in shallow portion of pool	1:15
H. Length of shallow portion of pool	14 feet
I. Length of upslope	15 feet
J. Distance at an overhead structure (indoor pool)	15 feet
K. Board length	8 feet
L. Length of pool	50 feet
M. Depth at start of transition, not less than	C minus 6 inches

FIGURE 12.3 Recommended diving envelope for all pools other than those designed to meet competitive diving rules.

Depth Markers

All residential pools should have depth markers on both the coping or edge of the deck of the pool, and on the interior wall of the pool above the water line. Figure 12.7 illustrates some depth markings that include no diving warnings.

Location of Pools

All pools should be located a minimum of 15 ft (20 ft is preferred) from any structure. This would prevent people from diving or jumping from roofs, balconies, trees, fences, and other adjacent structures into the pool. The motel shown in Figure 12.8 actually located part of the pool under a structure that created an invitation for people to jump or dive.

Warning Signs

All pools should have signs prohibiting diving where the water is less than 5 ft deep. The best location for signs is on the coping or edge of the pool. Additionally, the rules for all nondiving

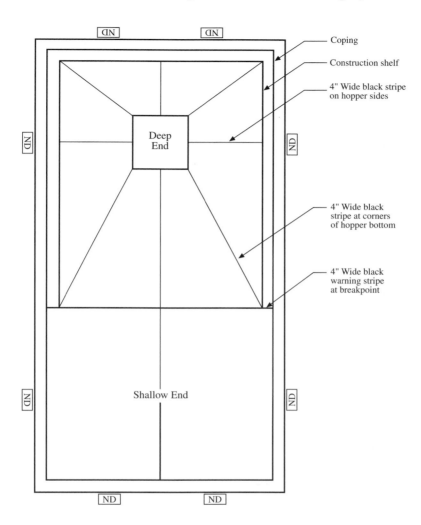

FIGURE 12.4 Recommended bottom markings for hopper-bottom pools.

pools should contain an item calling attention to the prohibition of diving. This prohibition of diving could be avoided if the sign we propose in our discussion of overcoming the dilemma in Chapter 15 is used (also see Chapter 13 on warning signs, and Appendix A).

LIGHTING

When swimming is to be permitted at night, the interior of the pool and the surrounding deck area must provide adequate lighting or night swimming should be prohibited.

POOL BARRIERS

All pools, including residential ones, should have a fence enclosing the facility to prevent intruders—particularly children—from having access; and gates must have positive, self-closing, and self-locking devices that children cannot open.

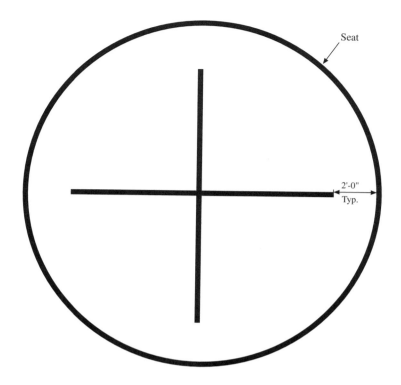

Seat

2'-0"
Typ.

FIGURE 12.5 Recommended bottom markings for round aboveground pools.

RECOMMENDATIONS FOR IMPROVING THE MANAGEMENT AND OPERATION OF POOLS

In addition to the need to change the design of pools, the Editorial Board believes that the way pools are regulated, managed, and operated must be improved. The recommendations follow.

SUPERVISION OF POOL PATRONS

All public and semipublic pools should have certified lifeguards—not merely attendants serving drinks and handing out towels—on duty at all times the facility is open see (Figure 12.9 and see Chapter 13). Owners of residential pools need to improve their knowledge of how to operate their pool safely and how to supervise their children and guests, and also need to learn cardiopulmonary resuscitation (CPR) and applicable swimming pool laws and regulations.

INDUSTRY STANDARDS

The standards promulgated by the National Spa and Pool Institute (NSPI) must address safety issues to a greater extent than they do at present. The NSPI membership relies on these standards in the design of their pools and in the preparation of their operating manuals.

STATE AND LOCAL LAWS AND REGULATIONS

All state and local rules and regulations governing public and semipublic pools should place greater emphasis on safety and should either publish separate regulations for residential pools or incorporate them in their public pool regulations in a separate section. Such matters as design, fencing, type of gates and locks, and covers for pools need to be conveyed to builders, manufacturers, and owners of residential pools.

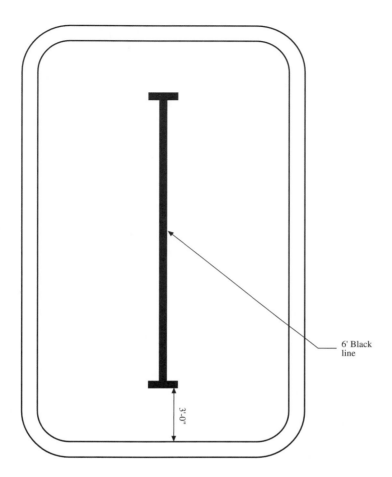

FIGURE 12.6 Recommended bottom markings for oval aboveground pools.

OTHER SPECIFIC RECOMMENDATIONS

The recommendations contained in this section are based not only on the data from this study but also on the years of experience of the members of the Editorial Board in consulting in the field of aquatics, writing about existing problems, and teaching thousands of youngsters and adults to swim and dive. The recommendations that follow go beyond the findings in this book and deal with overall problems associated with the safe operation of swimming pools. The recommendations are presented under the following categories:

- Correcting pool design defects
- Revising and strengthening pool standards and laws
- Improving the management and operation of semipublic and residential pools
- Strengthening communication with pool patrons

It is inevitable that some people considering these recommendations will ask, "How do you know they will reduce accidents?" The authors and Editorial Board do not—but based on the findings in this study and our many years of experience in aquatics, we strongly believe it is time to act now and evaluate the effectiveness of the changes as we go along. It would be careless—even reckless— to do nothing to combat the number of tragic injuries occurring to divers.

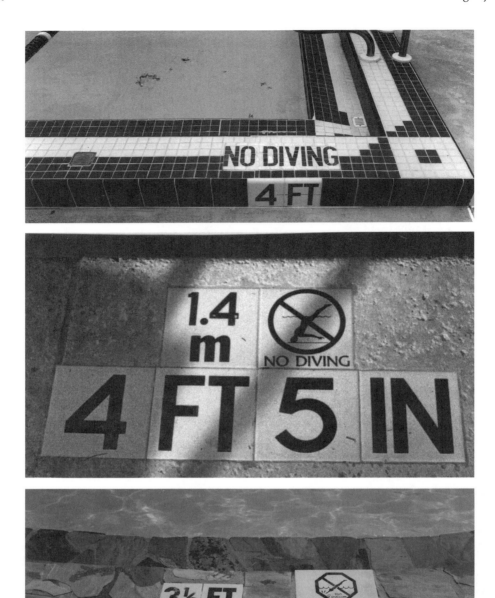

FIGURE 12.7 Depth markers not only indicate the depth of water in the pool but also can warn against diving where the water is too shallow for safety.

CORRECTING POOL DESIGN DEFECTS

Some authorities have concluded that there does not appear to be a need for a change in the way pools are designed or operated that will significantly reduce diving accident rates without adversely affecting the safety of others. While this position is apparently supported by the pool industry, it is emphatically rejected by the authors and the Editorial Board. In addition, we disagree that diving accidents are largely caused by errors on the part of the diver. In most cases the diver has not been found to be at fault. It is time that a critical examination is made of the way pools are designed, manufactured, sold, installed, operated, and supervised.

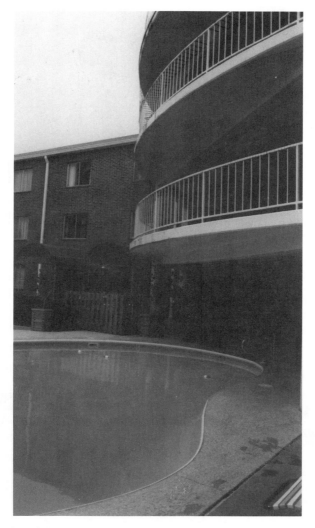

FIGURE 12.8 The portion of the pool under the balcony is an invitation for people to dive or jump.

Most diving injuries occur in the residential aboveground and inground "package pools". Consequently, manufacturers of these pools should carefully examine the findings and recommendations contained in this book. The following design recommendations, if implemented, will make pools safer for both swimming and diving. Making changes in existing pools may be difficult without "major surgery", nevertheless, many of the recommendations can be implemented without great cost to pool owners.

Water Depth of Pools

Shallow portion of pool

It is imperative that people understand that deep water (over people's heads) is where unknowing people usually drown, and that water less than 5 ft deep is where unknowing people usually break their necks from diving and become paralyzed for life.

In all pools other than wading or training pools, the depth of water in the shallow area must not be less than 3 ft. The depth of water in wading pools should range from 0 to 12 in. and in

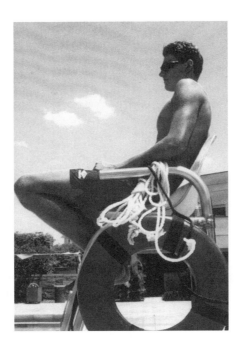

FIGURE 12.9 There is nothing better for ensuring the safety of pool patrons than the watchful eyes of a trained lifeguard.

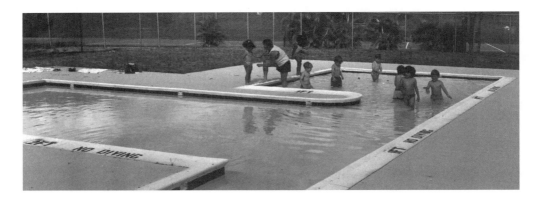

FIGURE 12.10   This is a pool for training children who cannot swim, which ranges in depth from 6 to 24 in.

training pools or sections, from 12 in. to $2\frac{1}{2}$ ft (Figure 12.10). These pools should be clearly identified with warnings as nondiving pools. The bottom of all pools other than aboveground and special-purpose pools should slope down at a ratio no greater than 1 ft vertical to 10 ft horizontal (1:10). Extending the shallow end of the pool out without a slope produces a constant depth area that should not be permitted because it creates a shallow shelf and a rapid, sharp drop-off of which first-time visitors will be unaware.

Diving envelope

For all pools with springboards or jumpboards—except those designed to meet the requirements of the ruling bodies of competitive swimming and diving such as the National Collegiate Athletic Association (NCAA), United States Diving (USD), National Federation of State High School

Athletic Associations (NFSHSAA), and International Swim and Dive Federation (FINA)—the bottom profile in the diving area should conform to the specifications shown in Figure 12.3.

We strongly recommend that there be only two pool standards for springboard diving. The first standard is for pools that are designed to meet the requirements for competitive diving; and the second standard is for all other pools with springboards or jumpboards—regardless of type—that are designed for recreational use. The basis behind this concept is that the diver will then have the same volume of water to pass through regardless of where he enters for the in-water trajectory. The specifications contained in Figure 12.3 were arrived at by research utilizing a variety of springboards and jumpboards, and subjects varying in size and athletic ability. See Appendix B for photos illustrating underwater trajectories. Pools that do not or cannot meet these specifications should be restricted to swimming with no diving equipment permitted or should restrict use to children under the age of 12.

Bottom Markings

Require bottom markings on all inground pools, regardless of size. All pools that do not have bottom racing lines, but have a diving well, should place a 6-in.-wide black stripe down the longitudinal axis in the center of the pool (Figure 12.11). A line should also be placed across the pool bottom at the "breakpoint" so that underwater swimmers can see it and it indicates where the deep water starts to the person planning to dive from the pool deck or springboard (Figure 12.12). It is essential that the person contemplating a dive, either from the deck or springboard, be able to see the bottom of the pool. When people are in, or have just exited the water, they invariably cause a disturbance of the water surface that makes it impossible to see the bottom because of reflections. Our solution is to place lines on the bottom of pools as shown in Figures 12.4 for hopper-bottom pools, in Figures 12.5 and 12.6 for aboveground pools, and in Figure 12.13 for internal steps and seats.

Depth Markings

Every pool should be required to have 6-in.-high depth markings located both at the edge of the deck (coping) and on the interior wall above the water line at every foot of change in water depth.

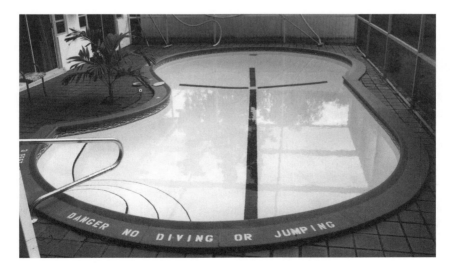

FIGURE 12.11 A line on the bottom of the pool along the longitudinal axis helps the potential diver to visualize the bottom contour of the pool.

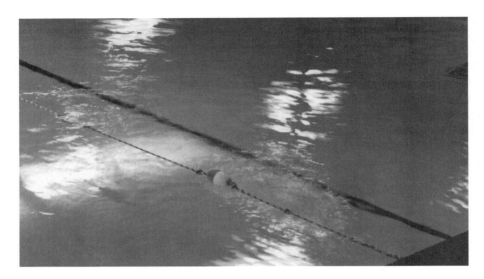

FIGURE 12.12 A lifeline across the surface of the pool at the breakpoint and a line on the bottom help people to see where the downslope of the pool starts. A lifeline at 1 to 2 ft in the shallow side provides a safety measure to discourage poor swimmers from getting into deep water.

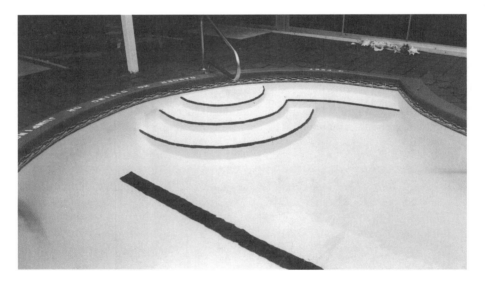

FIGURE 12.13 Recommended markings for internal steps and underwater seats.

Color of Pool Basin

The bottom of all pools should be white. So that the walls may be readily distinguished from the bottom, they should be colored light blue.

Coefficient of Friction of Bottom

The safe coefficient of friction of vinyl and painted pool bottom surfaces that should be employed in the bottom of pools needs to be established. There is considerable evidence that many of the diving injuries were the result of the hands slipping on the surface, thereby causing the head to be exposed to contact with the bottom.

Pool Location

All pools should be required to be located so that they are separated by at least 12 ft (preferably 15 ft) from any adjoining structure such as a garage, house, shed, balcony, tree, fence, and other objects that people may be tempted to use to dive or jump into the pool (see Figure 12.8).

Variable Depth Bottoms of Aboveground Pools

The practice of some aboveground pool manufacturers making pools with a variable depth available to customers should be discontinued. The added depth to the pool will encourage people to dive because they will interpret the added depth as an indication that it is safe for diving. In fact, this is not true. What can actually happen in these pools with variable bottoms is that the diver proceeds down the slope and strikes the upslope of the bottom.

Eliminate Hopper-Bottom Pools

Eliminate the construction of hopper-bottom pools. They are dangerously deceptive and constitute an entrapment to divers. Where hopper-bottom pools now exist, recommend to manufacturers and owners that the "seams" or "corners" be striped with a 4-in. black tape or paint to provide the diver with a discernible image of the pool bottom as shown in Figure 12.4.

Eliminate Spoon-Shaped Pool Bottoms

The spoon-shaped bottom profile in the diving portion (deep end) of inground gunite pools should be eliminated. It is dangerous for anyone diving from springboards or jumpboards because the maximum depth of water is at a single point, thus depriving the diver of a uniform safe diving area (see Figure 12.1 for proper diving envelope). The diver also cannot visualize the curvature of the sides with the bottom causing a deceptive image of the pool depth.

Eliminate Constant Depth in Shallow Portion of Pools

Eliminate the flat, constant depth portion of inground pools, usually found in vinyl-liner, hopper-bottom-type pools. This recommendation particularly applies to motel/hotel pools and some pools located at apartments/condominiums that attempt to incorporate an extensive area of shallow water in their pools to accommodate small children, most of whom are nonswimmers. Many of the diving injuries reported in this book were the result of people diving into the shallow portion of pools that had a constant depth of 3 ft.

Lighting for Night Swimming

Where pools are to be used for night swimming, a requirement of a minimum of 20 ft candles of illumination at the pool edge should be required, or diving at night should not be permitted. Where in-water lights are used, a minimum of 1.5 W/ft^2 of water surface area should be provided. It is essential for the diver to be able to see the bottom to ensure a safe dive.

Eliminate Safety Ledges

In construction of new pools, eliminate the so-called safety ledges (also referred to as "construction ledges") in the deep portion of pools. Where they now exist, we recommend that they be suitably marked (striped or colored) for easy identification. The ledge reduces the width of the pool underwater and serves as a walking ledge for youngsters, which has caused several drownings.

Mark Edges of Steps and Seats

Require that a black or dark blue edge be placed on the vertical and horizontal edge of all steps leading into the pool, and on the edge of underwater seats, as shown in Figure 12.13. As an alternative, finish the whole step in a contrasting color to make it more visible to those who may be contemplating a dive.

Recess All Steps and Ladders

Recess all steps and ladders into the pool wall with grab rails placed on the pool edge so that they do not extend into the water thereby causing an obstruction to swimmers and divers. Steps inserted into walls should be flush with no part protruding into the pool.

Recess Anchors and Receptacles

All anchors or receptacles for attaching lifelines and surface racing lines should be recessed into the wall so that they do not protrude into the pool and present a hazard to swimmers and divers.

Separate Spas and Hot Tubs

Spas and hot tubs should be separated from the pool by a distance of at least 20 ft to lessen the chance of people's getting out of the spa and immediately diving in the pool where the water might be too shallow. Spas should also be surrounded by a fence and have signs indicating rules for their use.

Lifeline

All pools that have a deep and shallow end should have a lifeline to identify the breakpoint (point where bottom starts to slope down toward deep end) (see Figure 12.12). The wall receptacles to which the lifeline is attached should be recessed 1 ft from the breakpoint toward the shallow end. This provides a visual reference to divers as to the specific location where the bottom starts to slope down.

Specify Location of Safe Diving Areas

Consideration should be given to coloring the coping or edge of pools "red" in those areas where diving from the deck of the pool is prohibited, and coloring the coping "green" where diving is permitted (see Figure 12.14). Diving from the deck should be prohibited for adults where the water is less than 5 ft deep, unless the pool incorporates the instructions we propose in Chapter 15.

Starting Blocks for Competitive Swimming

All starting blocks used for competitive swimming should be placed at the deep end of the pool unless the shallow end is more than 5 ft deep. In pools where this is not possible, starting blocks should be removed and races should be started from the deck. The competitive swimming ruling bodies (United States Swimming [USS], NCAA, and NFSHSAA) are urged to modify their rules to prevent the installation of starting blocks in any depth of water less than 6 ft. Where compliance with the rules is impossible, all swimming races should be started from the deck as opposed to starting blocks.

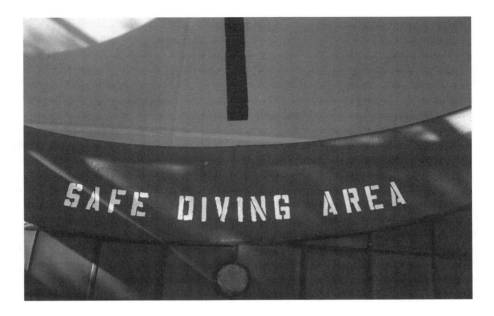

FIGURE 12.14 Illustration of marking on the coping, indicating safe diving area.

Depth Markers

Figure 12.7 shows types of depth markers, which include no diving warnings.

REVISING AND STRENGTHENING POOL STANDARDS AND LAWS

SWIMMING POOL INDUSTRY

Revision of NSPI Standards for Residential and Public Pools

The swimming pool industry (NSPI) needs to revise its standards with respect to the design of pools in accordance with the recommendations outlined in the previous section of pool design defects.

A summary of the needed revisions of the NSPI Standards for Residential Pools regarding pool design follows:

- Specifications for the diving envelope
- Hopper-bottom and spoon-shaped pools
- Location, content, and size of signs warning against diving in certain locations
- Specifications for pool bottom markings and markings on the edge of internal steps
- Specifications for boards including length, stand, and height above water

Recommendations for changes in the NSPI Standards for Public Pools include

- Correcting the specifications for the diving envelope
- Specifying the length and height of boards above the water, the extension of boards over the pool, and the type of stands for support of the board
- Requiring bottom markings for all pools indicating the size and location of the markings

- Requiring black edging on internal steps and seats
- Specifying the level of illumination for interior of the pool basin and the deck area

Recommendations concerning the operation of pools include:

- Requiring lifeguards for all semipublic pools
- Requiring fences and gates for all outdoor semipublic pools
- Specifying that owners and operators of apartment/condominium pools must not issue keys to renters or condominium owners to permit them to use the pool when it is closed
- Specifying the content and location of pool rules and signs warning against diving in certain locations

Manufacturers of Pools

Manufacturers of aboveground and package pools should have a section in their operating manuals dealing with the recommendations for the safe operation of the pool. Particular reference should be made to the steps that need to be taken for added protection when visitors use the pool or parties are held, requiring that greater emphasis be placed on the direct supervision of guests.

Fabricators of Pool Liners

Fabricators of pool liners for use in both aboveground and package inground pools should place depth markers on the liner above the water line and also lines on the bottom of the pool liner as indicated in Figures 12.5 and 12.6.

Manufacturers of Springboards/Jumpboards

Manufacturers of springboards/jumpboards must initiate a standards program followed by testing to establish the board efficiency and variation in human performance of divers with different physical characteristics. This is necessary as a means of establishing safe water depth and volume needed to accommodate the particular boards safely.

In the year 2000, there are practically no residential pools in the United States that can safely accommodate adults diving from springboards/jumpboards. The pools are too shallow and the upslope of the bottom starts too close to the end of the board. Furthermore, there are far too many different models and types of boards and stands being manufactured. The numbers must be reduced and boards must be tested by manufacturers to meet a new standard.

REGULATORY AGENCIES

State

The statutes enacted by states to govern public pools should be revised utilizing information contained in this book, particularly the recommendations for overcoming design defects outlined in a previous section. Particular attention must be given to changing the specifications of the deep end of the pool designed to accommodate diving from springboards/jumpboards.

The states, or the designated enforcers of the state regulations, should make certain that the pool "as built" conforms to the regulations of the state and to the plans as submitted for approval before granting the pool agency an operating permit. Many pools have been built that are different from filed plans.

Those local authorities, usually the county or major city designated by the state to enforce state regulations, should improve their inspections of pools, paying greater attention to the safety requirements established in the literature. States should make it mandatory that all public (and semipublic) pools provide qualified lifeguards at all times the facility is open.

States must not, in any way, make their laws less stringent for pools classified as semipublic, which are usually owned and operated by motels/hotels and apartments/condominiums. According to the findings presented in this book, the greatest number of spinal cord injuries as a result of diving occur in this pool classification when calculated on pool-to-user ratio.

Counties and Cities

The ordinances and building codes of counties and cities must be strengthened by incorporating essential safety features. They must specify the location parameters of pools in the backyard, the specifications for fencing around pools and yards, and other safety measures; code enforcement divisions should strictly enforce such codes.

Consumer Product Safety Commission

The Consumer Product Safety Commission (CPSC) holds a key position in the matter of pool safety. Among the steps they should be taking to elevate the level of pool safety are:

- Collecting data on diving accidents and establishing a standard data set and collection format
- Conducting or contracting to have conducted studies directed at determining human performance and physics related to pool design and diving equipment
- Holding meetings with state officials responsible for governing pools in their states to strive for greater uniformity
- Developing public service videotapes on pool safety and diving
- Monitoring standards developed by NSPI, American Public Health Institute (APHA), American National Standards Institute (ANSI), and ASTM
- Establishing a diving advisory committee consisting of coaches, divers, educators, researchers, architects, engineers, and public health department representatives to advise on the validity of published industry standards and new diving equipment.

IMPROVING THE MANAGEMENT AND OPERATION OF SEMIPUBLIC AND RESIDENTIAL POOLS

It must be realized that most diving injuries occur in pools located in motels/hotels, apartments/condominiums, and private residences. Of the 440 injuries reported on in this book, 365(83.0%) happened in these types of pools. One simple explanation is that these pools seldom have lifeguards and other qualified personnel supervising the patrons/guests, and their mode of operation and maintenance of the pools leaves much to be desired.

The authors and Editorial Board have these recommendations for pool owners to make their pools safer.

OWNERS OF RESIDENTIAL POOLS

- Supervise their children's use of the pool at all times.
- Make sure their children receive instruction in diving from a qualified instructor.
- Whenever guests are invited to use the pool, they must be supervised and, in particular, told what they cannot do and given the proper use of such equipment as diving boards, slides, and spas. Suggest to guests that they first enter the pool by going down steps or ladder and walk around to familiarize themselves with the facility.
- Place pool rules at every entrance and preferably on the gate itself.
- Check to be sure that the condition of the water is satisfactory. The bottom of the pool must be visible and clear of debris.

- Provide adequate lighting if the pool is to be used at night.
- Place slides at the deep end of the pool. No slides should be installed with aboveground pools.
- Place safety equipment where it can be reached quickly when needed.
- Instruct members of the household about the dangers associated with the use of the pool and suggest to teenagers that they take American Red Cross (ARC) courses in basic first aid, cardiopulmonary resuscitation (CPR), and water safety (community water safety course).
- Watch what the guests are doing and warn them if they are engaged in activities that are not permitted.
- Prohibit all diving in the shallow end of the pool or through an inner tube, hula hoop, or other floating devices.
- Learn all about how to maintain the pool properly by taking courses available locally or by retaining a qualified pool service company.
- Hire a lifeguard when planning a large party (over 25 people) where guests will be permitted to use the pool. Such a lifeguard can be hired by seeking qualified students from a local college or parks and recreation departments who are always looking for extra money.
- Place a safety cover on the pool when going away for a weekend or vacation to prevent neighbor children from gaining access.

OWNERS AND OPERATORS OF MOTEL/HOTEL, APARTMENT/CONDOMINIUM, AND ALL PUBLIC POOLS

- Lifeguards should be on duty whenever the pool is open.
- Secure the pool by locking fence gates or covering it when the pool is not open.
- Use TV monitoring of the pool when it is closed.
- Post rules at all entrances to the pool.
- Place signs prohibiting diving on the pool edge or coping where the water is less than 5 ft deep (see Figure 12.15).
- Install proper lighting if the pool is to be open after dark.
- Train pool operators to properly maintain the pool, to be familiar with state and local regulations, and to ensure compliance.
- Fence the pool area. Fences should be at least 5 ft high with 6 ft high preferred. All gates leading into the pool area must be locked (not just closed) whenever the pool is officially closed.

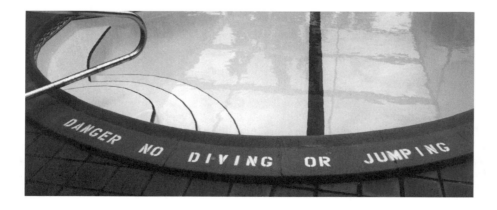

FIGURE 12.15 The best location for a sign prohibiting diving is on the coping, as shown in this photo.

STRENGTHENING THE COMMUNICATION WITH POOL PATRONS

The industry, pool owners, and operators must recognize that communication with pool users about safety and the dangers of diving in certain locations in the pool is essential; this can be accomplished through effective warning signs and by other means. Warnings placed at the pool are the last resort in preventing people from diving. Examples of warning signs are shown in Chapter 13. In addition to warning signs, rules for the use of the pool should be placed at all entrances of all facilities (see Appendix A).

SUMMARY

The Editorial Board's objective is to reduce the number of diving injuries occurring annually. In no way is this Board proposing the elimination of diving in swimming pools. If the recommendations set forth in this chapter are followed, the end result will be individuals diving into safer pools, and sustaining fewer broken necks.

Major efforts must be taken to educate the public about the dangers associated with diving into pools and the importance of safe diving in the prevention of spinal cord injury.

13 Warnings and Supervision: Essential Ingredients for Safety

INTRODUCTION

The authors and Editorial Board strongly believe that signs warning people about dangerous areas and activities are essential to the safety of potential users of facilities both in pools and in bodies of water in the natural environment. Signs are used to communicate important information to potential users of an aquatic facility concerning rules for its of use, existence of hazards, and ways to avoid personal injury. The communication of critical information about safety is a nondelegable responsibility of owners and operators of pools and other aquatic facilities and often can only be accomplished through the use of appropriately designed information signs.

PURPOSE OF WARNINGS

Signs accomplish the following three basic objectives:

1. To tell people about a threat to their well-being posed by dangerous conditions or products
2. To serve as a safety measure to change people's behavior so that they act safely (as opposed to acting unsafely)
3. To remind people of the first two objectives

If it is foreseeable that people can be injured when they act in a certain way, and careful evaluation shows that physical safety measures cannot be provided to ameliorate the consequences of persons' acts, then warnings to notify and remind those who are in danger are required. The existence of "open and obvious" hazards should not necessarily lead one to the conclusion that warnings are not needed, because reminding people about familiar hazards can prevent injuries. More likely, the danger of either risk or hazard is unsuspected and/or not obvious to the bather in the given circumstances. Warnings must be provided when known hazards remain as integral features of the swimming pool environment and human exposure to these hazards is possible. This remains true despite design efforts aimed at identifying and removing the hazards or reducing or eliminating the exposure.

WARNINGS IN PLACE OF SAFETY DESIGN MODIFICATIONS

An inventory of hazards needs to be systematically compiled and revised as appropriate by the pool designer, manufacturer, retailer, or owner and maintainers of the swimming pool facility. Categorization of swimming pool hazards is as follows:

Physical hazards

- Shallow water
- Internal stairs
- Deep water
- Springboards and diving towers
- Slippery surfaces
- Objects floating in the pool

Chemical hazards

- Chlorine gas
- Acid
- Liquid chlorine
- Chlorine-type granules
- Cleaning chemicals

Environmental hazards

- Lighting in and around the pool
- Cloudy water
- Algae
- Glare on surface from either low sunbeams or artificial light

Behavioral hazards

- Running
- Pushing people in the water
- Throwing people in the water
- Jumping on people
- Other forms of horseplay
- Unauthorized use of pools after hours
- Diving or jumping in water that is too shallow

Every pool owner and operator must catalog and analyze the hazards that exist within the pool environment. It is recommended that a formal, written analysis be prepared with each hazard unique to the facility listed. Beside each entry, the person performing the warning requirement analysis should identify possible methods for eliminating or mitigating the injurious conditions of the hazard or for protecting the user. Those hazards that remain on such a list and that cannot be eliminated or mitigated are candidates for warnings. Each must be evaluated to determine whether a warning might work or further effort can be made to eliminate, mitigate, or guard against the hazard.

Those hazards that survive this screening process must then be evaluated with respect to the intensity of the threat presented to the facility user. Warnings must be provided for all hidden hazards. The less obvious the hazard is, the more compelling the need to warn. On the other hand, the so-called obvious hazards may not be obvious to everyone, and certainly those that present a serious possibility of harm should be considered for reminder warnings. In general, if it is possible to anticipate that a warning may prevent an injury, it is appropriate to provide that warning. Warnings are necessary for important hazards because society has come to depend on the fact that hazards are always marked and that if no markings exist, the situation is safe.

EFFECTIVE WARNINGS

Warnings that successfully communicate a message and warnings that cause people to act safely have the following important characteristics in common:

1. Warnings attract attention to themselves by standing out distinctively from other features of the environment. Distinctive colors and shapes; the use of familiar signal words such as *danger, warning,* and *caution;* and the use of warning colors such as red, white, and black or black and yellow all serve to focus the attention of the people to be warned by the warning message. That is, effective warnings are designed to get attention.
2. Effective warnings are physically located in proximity to the actual hazard. In general, it is important to provide timely notice and reminder to those who must be warned. The greater the separation in time and place between the warning and the desired "safe" response, it is less likely that the response will be made.
3. Warnings provide motivation to act safely by explicitly stating the consequences of failure to act appropriately; the use of signal words *danger, warning,* and *caution* refer to the severity of the threat to the well-being of the person being warned. In this latter regard, the signal word *danger* is used to mark the possibility of serious, permanent injury or death; the signal word *warning* denotes the threat of serious recoverable injury; and the signal word *caution* is used to mark the possibility of moderate to minor injury.
4. Effective warnings clearly and concisely tell people how to avoid being hurt in a way that is readily understood and followed by those who are being warned. The consequences of *not obeying* the warning are unmistakably illustrated for the unsuspecting guest.
5. Warning signs must be durable, legible, illuminated, large in type, unambiguous, serious, and simply stated. See Figure 13.1 for illustrations of rules and warnings signs developed by motel and apartment pools.

STANDARDIZATION, PICTORIALS, AND TESTING

Using standardized warning formats (i.e., those in common use) increases the likelihood that the warning will be seen and promotes rapid recognition and surer adherence. (Refer to the American National Standards Institute (ANSI) publication.[1] The signal words *danger*, *warning*, and *caution* have standardized and well-known meanings. These signal words and the dangers they categorize are associated with color schemes that are equally well known (e.g., red, white, and black for *danger*; *orange* and black for *warning*; and yellow and black for *caution*). Similarly, warning signs are typically arranged in the signal word at the top (often in a standardized format such as the oval shape used with *danger*) and with a statement of the hazards and directions for avoiding injury. Deviations from these standardized formats should be carefully considered and well justified before being employed.

Pictorials, often referred to as graphics, present an opportunity to rapidly communicate the presence of a hazard or a behaviorally inappropriate action to the pool user without requiring written language familiarity. Simple, clear, clinically tested graphic warnings have a minimum use of any language; plus, universally understood symbols are most preferable.

New, never-tried warnings need to be tested carefully for meaning, recognition, and potentially dangerous misinterpretation. The use of focus group interviews conducted by experienced clinical psychologists or safety experts using relatively simple market-testing methods is appropriate for the evaluation of new warnings. At the very least, a new sign should be shown to a representative sample of unsophisticated swimmers (20 or more) for comment to ensure that the intended meaning is communicated and dangerous reversals of meaning do not occur. Clearly, if even one dangerous misinterpretation in a group of 20 is discovered, the warning design effort must be repeated.

LOOK Before you LEAP!

POOL RULES
1. Swim at your own risk
2. Hotel guests only - Proper I.D. required
3. No running or rough play
4. One person on diving board at a time
5. Straight diving only - No fancy dives
6. No diving from pool edges - Use diving board only
7. Glass not permitted in this area
8. Shirts and shoes required in lobby and restaurant
9. Hours: 9:00 a.m to 9:00 p.m.

OUR POOL RULES

USE BATHROOM NOT OUR POOL

GO EASY ON HAIR & SKIN OIL

BEST NOT SWIM ALONE

NO UNNECESSARY NOISE   NO ROUGH PLAY

LADIES! PLEASE WEAR CAPS!

DON'T DIVE INTO SHALLOW END

POOL RULES
Pool Hours 8 am - 10 pm
NO DIVING

NO
- Lifeguard on duty. Swim at your own risk
- Diving, running or horseplay in pool area
- Diving gear or rafts in pool
- Glass containers in pool area
- Alcoholic beverage in pool area
- Cut offs, swim suit only

Children must be accompanied by an adult
Registered guest only -Trespasser prosecuted

- Swim at your own risk
- Children must be acompanied by an adult
- Registered guests only
- No glass containers allowed
- Keep off divider rope

POOL RULES
- No animals in pool or on pool deck
- No food or drink in pool or within four feet of pool
- Shower before entering pool
- Bathing load 65 persons at one time
- Pool hours: 9 am to 5 pm

NO DIVING
(Unless you have an approved diving bowl)

- Location of nearest telephone for emergency use: Cabana Office
- Maximum temperature for use is 105°F

WARNING! NO LIFEGUARD ON DUTY
1 • All persons using pool do so at own risk. Management is not responsible for accidents or injuries, lost or stolen property
2 • Residents only - Guests must have prior permission from manager
3 • Children under 16 years must be accompanied by an adult and supervised at all times
4 • No running, jumping or horseplay in or around the pool area
5 • Diving prohibited
6 • No glass of any kind in the pool area
7 • No pets or wheeled vehicles in or around pool
8 • Excessive noise not permitted at any time
9 • Management reserves the right to deny use of pool to anyone at any time
10 • Pool Hours 10 a.m. – sunset

FIGURE 13.1 Warning signs and pool rules that have been used by many motels and hotels.

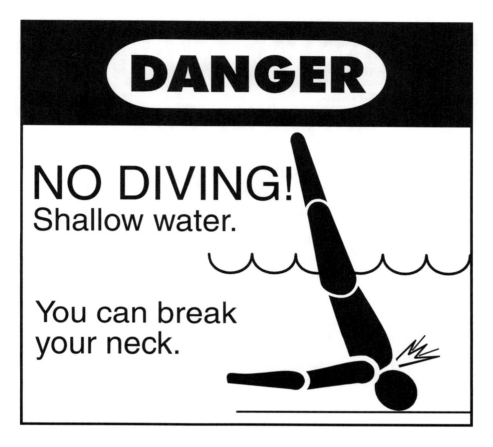

FIGURE 13.2 This is the sign that the American Institute for Research (AIR) recommended to be used to prevent diving injuries.

OTHER STUDIES RELATIVE TO WARNING SIGNS

In 1985, the National Swimming Pool Foundation (NSPF) contracted with the firm of Dorris and Associates to conduct a study on signs for pools and spas. The report clearly supported the need for warning signs in swimming pools.[2]

Then in 1988, the American Institute for Research (AIR) under contract with the U.S. Consumer Product Safety Commission (CPSC) conducted a study, including a detailed evaluation of 22 existing warning signs provided to them by CPSC.[3] Figure 13.2 is the sign recommended by them to prevent diving injuries. Figures 13.3 and 13.4 depict other signs prohibiting diving.

WARNINGS SUMMARY

Warnings are required when hidden hazards exist or continue to exist despite engineering and other efforts to either eliminate or reduce the injurious potential of the hazard or to guard people from coming into contact with the hazard. The hazards at a facility should be systematically evaluated to determine the likely candidates for warnings. Warnings should be developed in standardized formats to promote rapid recognition and to maximize adherence. Mechanically, warnings should be legible, understandable, serious in tone, and durable. Warnings should be tested. Well-designed, carefully thought out warnings can add considerable safety because they help control the critical behavioral

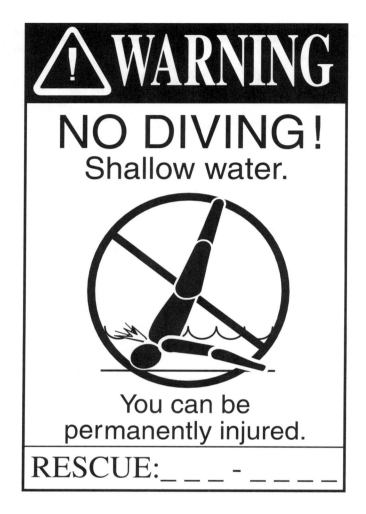

FIGURE 13.3 This is the sign that the National Swimming Pool Foundation (NSPF) produced.

element involved in every facility-related injury. Also, manufacturers of aboveground and prefabricated inground pools should place appropriate warnings directly on their pools at the assembly plant.

GUIDELINES FOR POOL OWNERS

- All pubic and semipublic pools should employ qualified and certified lifeguards to supervise patrons whenever the pool is open for use. The posting of a sign by owners stating, "No lifeguard on duty—swim at your own risk" is unreasonable and unacceptable.
- The decision of many owners of motels/hotels and apartments/condominiums not to provide lifeguards is a serious mistake. Few drownings would ever occur if, when the pool is open for operation, a certified lifeguard was on duty. To provide a lifeguard for a pool located at a 200-room motel would add no more than 50 cents to the room rate, which in 2000 figures ranges from $40 to more than $100. Few, if any, patrons would object to paying an additional 50 cents. It is the opinion of the Editorial Board that states must mandate the staffing of all public pools with certified lifeguards.

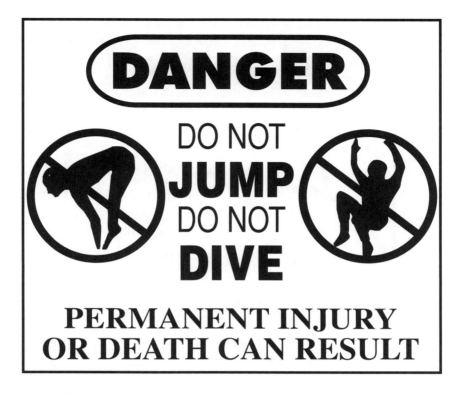

(a)

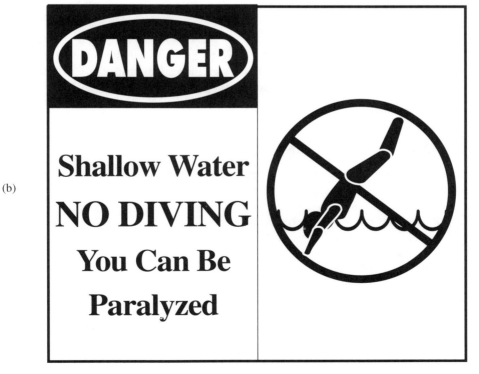

(b)

FIGURE 13.4 These are other signs that have been used since 1980.

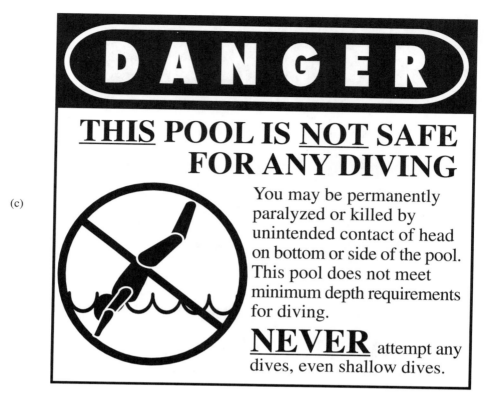

(c)

FIGURE 13.4 (Continued)

- Owners of residential pools should seek or be given instructions on how to supervise their children and guests who swim and dive there. This instruction can be provided in a booklet prepared by the pool industry, by professional individuals, or by aquatic organizations.

TYPICAL OBJECTIONS TO SIGNS

Confronting the industry and regulatory agencies has been the intense outcry from pool owners, builders, manufacturers, and the public saying:

- "I do not want my pool cluttered up with signs."
- "Signs have not proven to be effective in reducing the number of diving injuries—why do we need them?"
- "People do not obey signs."
- "Signs only encourage people to do just the opposite."
- "Authorities overestimate the importance of signs."
- "Kids only tear signs down; they do not obey them."
- "Signs around backyard pools detract from the kind of atmosphere desired in a family setting."
- "Signs do not help me sell pools!" (pool manufacturer)

Despite these objections, warning signs are an essential component of aquatic safety.

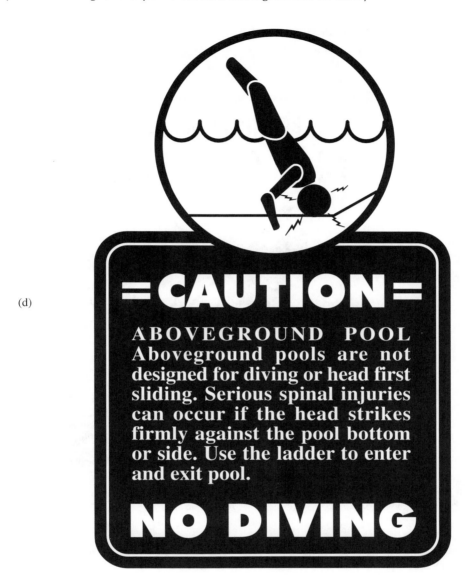

(d)

FIGURE 13.4 (Continued)

RESPONSIBILITY TO POST SIGNS

Who has the responsibility to see that signs are provided for pools? Our recommendations follow:

- **Industry**—The pool industry (National Spa and Pool Institute [NSPI]) should include in its standards recommending the need for warning signs including location, content, and rules for the pool. It should also develop and make available to its members the kinds of signs appropriate for various types of pools and activities.
- **Manufacturers**—Manufacturers of pools should acquire signs from NSPI or develop their own signs and place them on the pools before they leave their plant.

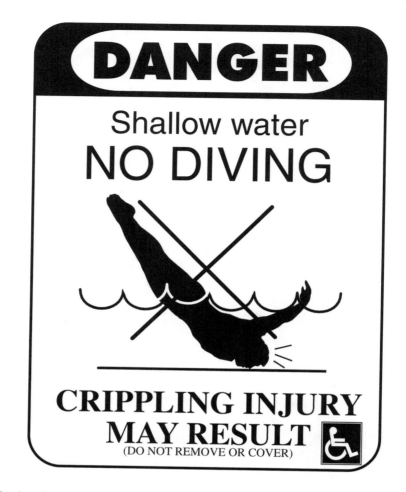

(e)

FIGURE 13.4 (Continued)

- **Architects and engineers**—Architects and engineers who design pools should specify the kinds of signs needed and their location, and provide them either to customers or the contractor with instructions for installation.
- **Owners**—Owners of pools must be prepared to replace signs that are torn down, are vandalized, or have faded to the extent that they are not legible. Owners of motels/hotels and apartments/condominiums that provide pools for their guests/tenants have, in addition to the posting of signs in the pool area, the responsibility to communicate specific safety information pertaining to the use of the pool. These instructions should be posted in every motel/hotel room and also could actually be given to guests as they register or to each new apartment/condominium resident. An example of such instructions for use with motels/hotels is contained in Appendix A.

SIGNAGE FOR USE ADJACENT TO NATURAL BODIES OF WATER

Owners and managers of land that contains lakes, rivers, creeks, canals, ocean embayments, and reservoirs have a duty to warn users of their land where dangerous and hazardous water conditions exist or might exist. This includes individuals and governmental agencies at all levels, from villages to departments of the federal government, such as the Army Corps of Engineers and the National Park Service. Some of the dangerous areas and conditions that have resulted in injuries or death to people who are seeking fun and recreation in the outdoors are:

- Cliffs adjoining rivers and lakes
- Underwater obstructions such as stumps, rocks, and deadheads
- Man-made retaining walls or bulkheads along shores of rivers and lakes
- Docks or piers extending out into rivers, lakes, and the ocean
- Holes or drop-offs in the beach areas
- Sandbars usually found in rivers and ocean beaches
- Settings created by natural forces such as heavy surf, rip currents, rapids, and other water movement
- Bridges over rivers and creeks
- Rope chains or cables attached to trusses used by youngsters to swing out into rivers and lakes
- Banks or ledges of quarries
- Jetties extending into lakes or the ocean
- Dams and waterfalls
- Water discharge from plants (electrical, manufacturing, and nuclear)
- Structures such as motels/hotels, sheds, or warehouses located next to rivers or lakes where youngsters are tempted to dive or jump from their roofs or balconies

Warnings in the settings described may utilize one or more of the following approaches:

- Warning signs placed on or near the hazard
- Rules for use of waterways, placed on water vehicles such as boats, rafts, and canoes
- Safety booklets at entrance to parks
- Posted rules at swimming beaches stating proper use and prohibited activities

Rivers do not need signs posted every 100 yards. Only after an assessment has been made of where people are entering, stopping to participate in swimming and diving in some of the settings cited earlier, and leaving the river should warnings be posted at these locations.

GUIDELINES FOR OWNERS OF NATURAL WATER AREAS

Listed next are requirements the Editorial Board believes are needed relative to supervision of people in designated water areas in the natural environment:

- All designated swimming beaches should be staffed with an adequate number of qualified lifeguards.
- When lifeguards go off duty, the beach or swimming area should be closed and signs should be posted to that effect.
- All boating, canoeing, sailing, water skiing, scuba diving, and other special activities need to be managed and operated by people who are qualified in the activity. This includes those that are operated by concessionaires.
- At locations on rivers and lakes where people are permitted to launch boats, there should be a sign posted indicating what the regulations are relative to the use of the area and its waters.
- When churches, schools, colleges, scouts, hospitals, and other community agencies are sponsors of groups for picnics, campouts, or just a recreational outing at or near waters, there are two essential steps that they must take. First, they should determine what

supervision, such as lifeguards will be available at the destination. Second, they should decide what supervision they must provide to ensure the safety of the participants. In some cases, it may be necessary for them to hire qualified people to supervise specific activities.

IS SUPERVISION NECESSARY? THE ANSWER IS YES!

After addressing the importance of well-designed and executed warning signs, some may ask whether supervision is still necessary. The extent to which people need to be supervised when engaged in aquatic activities has been debated for years. Based on research and extensive years of combined experience in aquatics, the authors and Editorial Board believe the answer is yes. In our opinion, there is no better way to prevent drownings or serious injuries than to have someone who is qualified in aquatic safety and lifesaving in a position to watch, supervise, and control the activities of swimmers and divers.

REFERENCES

1. American National Standards Institute,
2. National Swimming Pool Foundation (NSPF), Precautionary Information for Swimming Pools and Spas: Consumer Preference and Understanding, Dorris & Assoc., 1986.
3. U.S. Consumer Product Safety Commission (CPSC), Existing and Proposed Warning Messages for Signs that May be Posted at Swimming Pools, American Institute for Research (AIR), Contract CPSC-C-86-1163, 1988.

14 A Coach Looks at the Data

At the request of the authors of this book, I have reviewed the data concerning diving injuries and was literally shocked when it became evident that most of these injuries should not have happened. Why did they happen? The answer was quite clear. It was the failure of those who design, operate, and maintain pools; and those who develop the standards and regulations governing the specifications of the diving envelope by which the pools were constructed.

Diving is, without a doubt, the most exciting and fun activity that both kids and adults can do in a pool. When diving, they literally fly through the air, enter the water headfirst, and return to the surface.

My life's work has primarily been in competitive diving—from springboard to platform diving. However, I have taught many children and adults to dive from boards and decks of pools who were not competitive divers. We are all indebted to the work of R. Jackson Smith, a former diving champion, and an outstanding architect who back in the 1950s developed the specifications for the diving envelope for pools designed to accommodate both springboard and platform competitive diving. Because of his work no one has ever broken his neck by hitting the bottom of pools that conform to his specifications. This includes recreational divers using the competitive diving equipment. Using his specifications as a reference, International Swim and Dive Federation (FINA, the international governing body for competitive diving) adopted new specifications for competitive diving. These specifications have also been adopted by United States Diving (USD), the National Collegiate Athletic Association (NCAA), and the National Federation of State High School Athletic Associations (NFSHSAA). Table 14.1 contains the FINA specifications for 1-m boards. The noncompetitive diving pools are guided by regulations promulgated by states for both public and semipublic pools. States do not publish standards for residential pools. The National Spa and Pool Institute (NSPI) has developed standards for both pubic and residential pools.

Today, most major pool facilities separate the diving envelope from the competitive swimming pool (Figure 14.1). In addition, competitive divers have coaches who instruct them in the proper diving mechanics including safe underwater trajectories. Few people understand that, in fact, practically none of the competitive divers go to the bottom of the pool. They either rotate or scoop up once they are underwater. They are taught to do this on all types of dives, from 1 and 3-m springboards and from all platforms up to 10 m in height.

TABLE 14.1
FINA Specifications for 1-m High Board

Dimension	m	ft / in.
Height of board above water	1.00	3/3 3/8
Depth of water at plummet	3.40	11/1 7/8
Distance from board to upslope	5.00	16/4 7/8
From plummet back to pool wall	1.80	5/10 7/8
Plummet to wall at side	2.00	6/6 6/8
From plummet to wall ahead	9.00	29/6 3/8

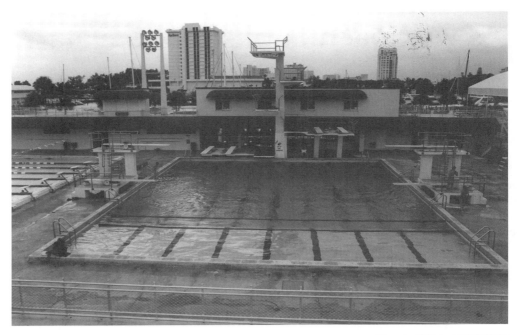

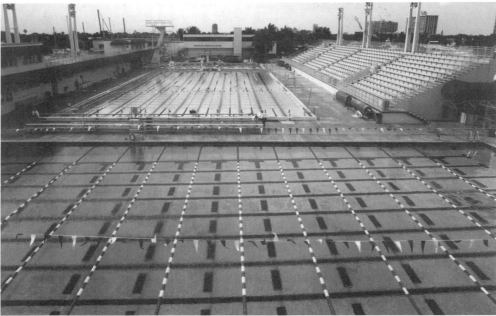

FIGURE 14.1 Photos of pools at International Swimming Hall of Fame: top, diving complex; bottom, two 50-m competitive pools.

OBSERVATIONS CONCERNING RECREATIONAL AND COMPETITIVE DIVERS

Competitive diving facilities are frequently open to everyone and it is frightening to see what lack of control some recreational divers have from the 1 and 3-m springboards. Fortunately, none have been injured as a result of hitting the bottom, due to R. Jackson Smith's influence on making these pools deep enough to accommodate any kind of dive.

Recreational divers performing from competitive springboards sometimes do "crazy dives," as shown in Figure 14.2. Some daredevils try jumping off a 10-m platform and many do stunts. Few get hurt, other than a slap on the back or stomach, because they never go deep enough to strike the bottom.

Others just try to make a simple dive from the 1- and 3-m boards. Wrong moves that many make when diving off the 1- and 3-meter boards include:

- They bounce on the end of the board.
- They run instead of walking to the end of the board and take off on one foot.
- They try dives for which they have been given no instruction.

The untrained recreational diver, because of lack of instruction, is apt to put himself in trouble, as shown in Figure 14.3 where he entered the water 13 ft from the board at an entry angle of 45 degrees. This was due to angle of takeoff, as shown in Figure 14.4. An athletic person can project himself as high above the board and out into the pool as shown in Figure 14.5.

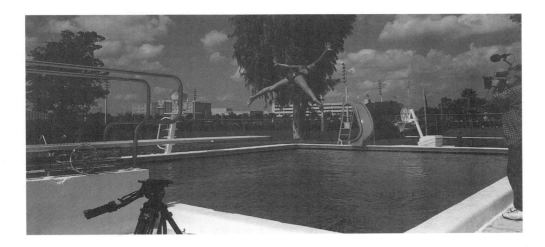

FIGURE 14.2 An example of a "crazy dive" made by a recreational diver.

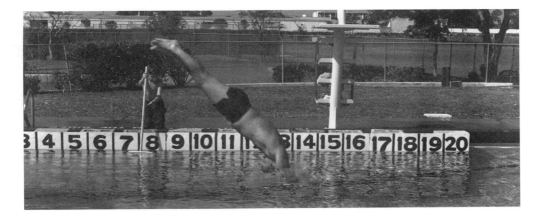

FIGURE 14.3 Entry angle and point recreational diver can achieve from a dive off a 6-ft-long jumpboard (12 ft out and 45 degree angle of entry).

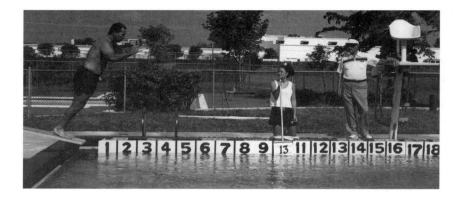

FIGURE 14.4 Recreational diver leaning forward on takeoff from board projects himself out a considerable distance.

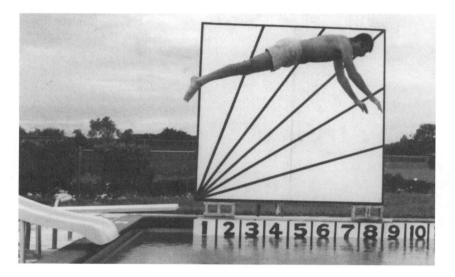

FIGURE 14.5 Indicates the height a recreational, athletic diver can obtain from an 8-ft-long springboard (26 in. above the water).

There is a correct way to dive, as indicated by competitive divers shown in the following figures. In Figure 14.6 the diver demonstrates the correct hurdle to the end of the board. Figure 14.7 illustrates the board depression, which gives the diver the spring to thrust himself upward. Figure 14.8 shows the height above the board achieved by a good competitive diver. Trained competitive divers always enter the water close to the vertical, as shown in Figure 14.9. Competitive divers once underwater usually interrupt their vertical body alignment by rolling over or scooping up by arching their backs, raising their heads up, and pushing down with their hands. Figure 14.10 shows that a competitive diver holding his vertical body alignment can go down as deep as 18 ft.

Diving into shallow water (4 ft and less) causes more injuries than dives made from springboards. Actions divers take that can lead to injury when diving from the deck of the pool include:

- They fail to plan the dive, and instead perform an impulsive dive.
- They run to the edge of the pool and take off from one foot.
- They attempt to make a high jackknife dive.
- They enter the water at too steep an angle.

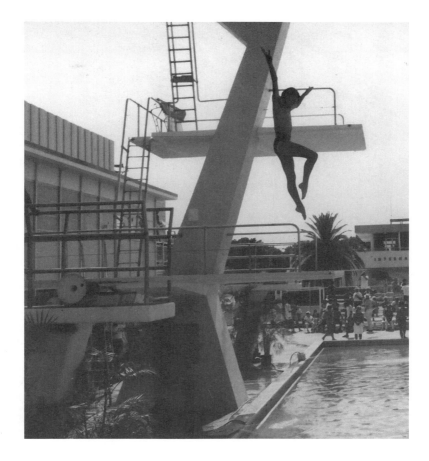

FIGURE 14.6 Competitive diver performing hurdle to end of 3-m-high springboard.

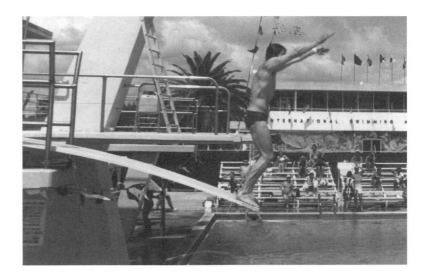

FIGURE 14.7 Depression of board by competitive diver, which produces the height diver achieves, as shown in Figure 14.5.

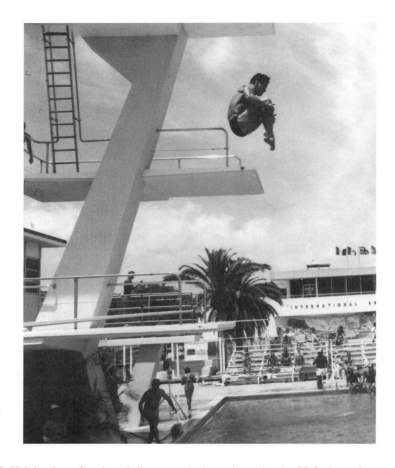

FIGURE 14.8 Height above 3-m board diver can obtain, estimated to be 20 ft above the water.

- They may flex the head down below the arms.
- They hold the arms too high above their heads.
- They attempt to dive through someone's legs or through a tube or hula hoop.
- They are unaware of the short time interval between entering the water and possible contact with the bottom (see Chapter 10 for the mechanics of diving).

FINDINGS AND IMPLICATIONS OF DATA
FROM THE 440 DIVING CASES

I have studied the data presented in this book (Chapters 4 to 8) relative to the 440 dives into swimming pools that caused spinal cord injuries to the diver. My findings and the implications of each follow:

1. In 336(76.4%) of the 440 cases, there was no qualified lifeguard on duty at the pool at the time the victim was injured. The implication of this is very simple. A lifeguard's responsibility is to prevent accidents from happening and, in my opinion, many of these injuries would not have occurred if a lifeguard or someone qualified in pool safety had been present.
2. In 337(76.6%) of the injuries, the depth of water where the victim struck the bottom was 4 ft or less with most less than $3\frac{1}{2}$ ft. The implication is that diving into shallow water is potentially dangerous unless you have been taught how to make a safe shallow dive.

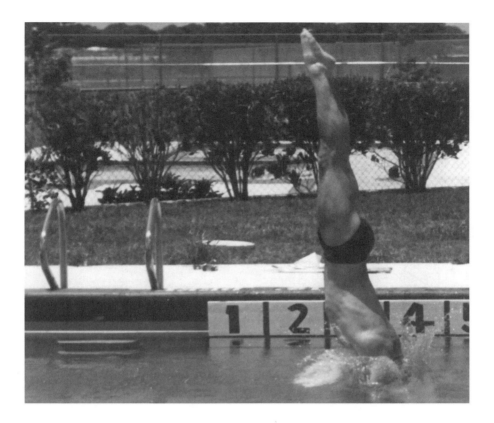

FIGURE 14.9 Angle of entry of trained diver.

3. The 32(7.3%) injuries to competitive swimmers as a result of diving off starting blocks should never have happened and will not in the future because the governing bodies for competitive swimming acted quickly to require deeper water or to lower the height of the starting blocks. The implications were that water $3\frac{1}{2}$ ft deep was not deep enough for a beginner (junior and senior high school swimmers) to learn the dive starts from blocks. The coaches made the mistake of not placing a starting block in the deep end of the pool where beginners could practice their starts.

4. In every one of the 92 injuries (Chapter 7) resulting from dives off springboards or jumpboards, the victim struck the upslope of the pool bottom. None hit at the deepest point of the pool; even in the 15 dives off 3-m-high boards, the victim hit the upslope of the bottom. The implications are that pools designed to accommodate diving from a board not only must be deeper but also must have the start of the upslope farther from the end of the board. See Chapter 12 for the specifications for safe diving envelope for all pools that are not of the competitive type.

5. The injuries of 273(62.0%) victims occurred on the first visit they made to the accident pool. The implications are that the victims were unaware of the existing pool conditions that were potentially hazardous and subsequently were extremely dangerous. Very little effort had been made to call to the attention of guests that diving was not permitted in the specific location where they made their dive. Again, the victims were not properly warned (see Chapter 13 on the importance of warnings).

6. Some form of alcoholic beverage, mostly beer, had been consumed by 179(40.7%) of the victims before they made their fateful dives. Again, the implication is clear that the

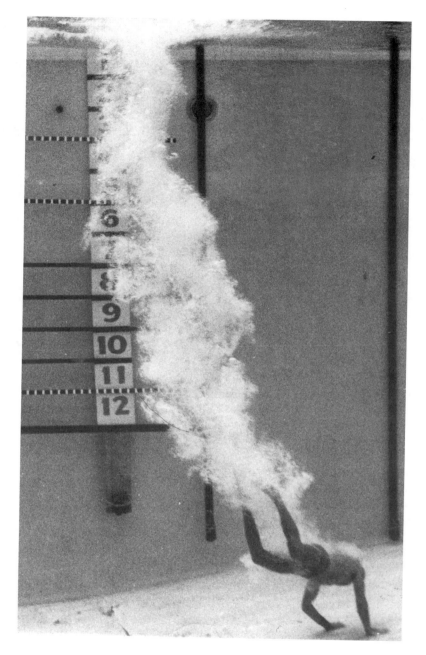

FIGURE 14.10 A competitive diver striking the bottom of pool 18 ft deep from dive off 10-m tower.

victims had not been told by anyone that they should not dive, and none of the signs warned against diving after drinking alcoholic beverages.

7. A most significant fact revealed by the data was that only 13 (3.0%) of the victims were members of the household that owned the pool. This implies that direct supervision of guests invited to swim in the pool is essential, that warning signs are necessary to convey to guests the existence of potential dangers, and that diving is not permitted in certain locations in the pool.

TABLE 14.2
Rules for Use of the Spring Board or Jump Board

Before using the diving board, familiarize yourself with the pool
- Get in and walk around on the bottom.
- Locate the breakpoint.
- Check the depth of the water.

Then follow these rules
- Plan your dive—know what you have to do to make your dive safe.
- Check the depth of water in front of the board.
- On the first dives, do a standing jump into the pool; then take a standing dive from the end of the board.
- Keep your arms in front on entry with the head between the arms.
- Do not double bounce on the board.
- Dive only straight out, never off the side of the board.
- Only one person at a time should be on the board.
- Be sure the diver preceding you is clear before you dive.
- Do not run on the board and take off on one foot—this will increase your entry velocity and may cause you to go out too far.
- After entry, arch your back and raise your head to return to the surface.
- On returning to the surface, immediately proceed to the side of the pool.
- Never attempt to jump or dive through hula hoops or inner tubes.
- Do not try crazy stunts like sailor's dives or any other horseplay on the board.
- Do not attempt dives for which you have had no professional instruction.
- Do not dive if you have been drinking or have used any drugs.
- Do not dive off the board if you are significantly overweight.

8. In 215 (48.9%) of the cases, the pools had no rules or signs posted to tell visitors where it was safe to dive or to forbid diving. The implication of this is that all owners and operators of pools must make every effort to convey to potential pool users how they must conduct themselves when using the pool. Again, this is best accomplished through proper communication with pool users as outlined in Chapter 13.

9. In 372 (84.5%) of the cases, the pools had no specific signs posted stating that diving was prohibited. A properly worded and placed sign saying, "Diving is not permitted in this pool," is imperative if the pool is too shallow, and represents the last opportunity to communicate with the potential diver.

To ensure the safe use of diving boards, it is essential to have rules near the board. Table 14.2 indicates what I consider to be an effective and appropriate set of rules to guide people attempting to use a springboard or jumpboard.

CONCLUSIONS

Most diving accidents into pools can be avoided if the pool patrons are forewarned relative to where and where not to dive, are informed about the correct way to dive, and are given the rules to dive safely (see Chapter 15). This can be accomplished by a combination of easily readable, well-placed warning signs in all pools and the presence of qualified people to supervise and control the diving activities of pool users. See Chapter 13 on warnings and supervision, and Figure 14.10 on how deep competitive divers can go if they fail to roll over or scoop.

Finally, I agree that diving in pools should not be prohibited. I also concur with the recommendations for safe diving from the deck of pools as set forth in Chapter 15, Figure 15.1a. All owners and operators of pools must make every effort to inform and supervise their guests if the number of diving injuries are to be reduced.

15 The Dilemma: The Controversial Issue of No Diving

What has the research concerning the 601 diving injury cases indicated that needs to be done to reduce the number of diving injuries occurring in swimming pools and in the water areas located in the natural environment? In Chapter 12 we made our recommendations for improving the design and operation of pools as well as the strengthening of standards, regulations, and laws. We have reached several conclusions as to the actions that are needed if the number of diving injuries is to be reduced. Before citing them we discuss the implications of our findings.

WHAT ARE THE IMPLICATIONS OF THE FINDINGS?

What do the data contained in this book really tell us? What are the implications? Some people have already overreacted to the diving problem. Others do not know what to do. Some families are now questioning whether they should buy a pool or not. Others are uncertain about installing a diving board or slide in their pools. We have considered many of the questions raised by government officials, concerned citizens, aquatic professionals, and the pool industry. We offer our answers to some of the following more disturbing questions:

- Does this literally mean the end to all diving into pools other than those strictly designed for diving? No.
- Does it mean that adults will be denied the thrill of diving from decks of residential pools? No.
- Does it mean that, as a nation, we have to accept the fact that 200 or 300 people each year will become quadriplegics as a result of diving into pools, or that another 400 to 500 will become quadriplegics as a result of diving into bodies of water located in the natural environment? No.
- Does it mean people should not be buying pools for their backyards? Emphatically, no.
- Does it mean that motels and hotels should stop offering pool facilities to their guests? No.
- Does it mean that developers should stop including swimming pools as one of the recreational activities provided to their tenants/owners? No.
- Does it mean that pool must be designed safer? Yes.
- Does it mean that all who own pools must operate and maintain them in a more efficient and safer manner? Yes.
- Does it mean that all public pools including apartments/condominiums and motels/hotels should have certified lifeguards on duty at all times that the pools are open? Yes.
- Does it mean that all pools—both residential and public—must have effective signage that conveys to users essential safety information? Yes.
- Does it mean that the swimming pool industry has been derelict in its responsibility to its members by failing to incorporate essential safety information in its standards? Yes.

- Does it mean that state laws and regulations governing pools are deficient with respect to safety? Yes.
- Does it mean that states must establish regulations or some type of guidance for the design, operation, and maintenance of residential pools? Yes.
- Does it mean that agencies and individuals who have the responsibility for teaching people to swim and dive must expand their instructional mode to include greater emphasis on how to dive safely and where to dive? Yes.
- Does it mean that the news media must become involved to a much greater extent in informing the public concerning what constitutes safe swimming and diving areas and what precautions must be taken to avoid injury? Yes.
- Does it mean that schools need to teach students about where to swim and dive, how to execute safe dives, and what the dangers are of mixing alcohol or drugs with swimming and diving? Yes.
- Does it mean that springboards or jumpboards probably should be removed from some pools? Yes.
- Does it mean that manufacturers are producing too many different sizes and models of springboards, jumpboards, and stands? Yes.
- Does it mean that more and better directed research on springboard/jumpboard diving is needed to incorporate variations in human performance in relation to different physical characteristics, board sizes, designs of stands, and heights of boards off the water, and profiles of pool bottoms? Yes.
- Does it mean that anyone contemplating a dive should know what he is diving into by direct examination of the pool or by inquiry as to the conditions? Yes.
- Does it mean that divers should enter the pool or any other body of water feet first if they have never been to the pool or area before? Yes.
- Do pool manufacturers, builders, distributors, and retailers need to do a better job of communicating safety information to customers? Yes.
- Does it mean that owners of residential pools need to provide better supervision of their guests when they or their children invite them to come for a swim? Yes.
- Does it mean that all pools must have posted in a conspicuous location rules for the use of the pool, other signs designed to warn people where they must not dive, and the consequences stated if they should choose to dive? Yes.
- Is it true that pools are the safest place to swim and that fewer people are injured from diving into pools than into other bodies of water? Yes.

While pools, in our opinion, are the safest places to swim, they still have the potential to be devastatingly dangerous.

RECOMMENDED ACTIONS

There are several areas where we believe action must be taken if we are to reduce the number of these catastrophic diving injuries. The task will not be easy and will require effort and cooperation on the part of many individuals and both public and voluntary agencies. We therefore recommend that all those involved in any way with designing, building, operating, and owning pools need to carefully study and then take these positive actions.

EDUCATE THE PUBLIC

The most important step involves educating the public. The quadriplegic victims interviewed were ignorant of the potential dangers associated with diving. They simply did not believe or know that they could break their necks doing what they did.

Any education program related to diving must be nationwide and directed at all ages: children, teenagers, and adults. Special effort must be made to distribute safety information to owners, operators, manufacturers, distributors, and installers of pools. If a school program could be initiated whereby, in the spring semester prior to the summer swimming season, every child would be exposed to films or verbal presentations on the dangers associated with diving, we believe fewer accidents would occur in the aquatic environment. Some suggestions for meeting this educational need follow.

Video Tapes

Prepare a variety of videotapes for use to educate owners, operators, and patrons of swimming pools relative to their responsibility in maintaining, operating, and using the facility safely. Among those to whom the tapes should be directed are

- Families who own or plan to buy a swimming pool
- Owners and operators of motel/hotel pools
- Operators of apartment/condominium pools
- School administrators and teachers for use in classrooms
- City and voluntary agency supervisors who conduct swimming programs in pools
- Local and network television outlets, advertisers, and broadcasters

Who should assume the responsibility for preparing these tapes? We believe these agencies or organizations could, and should, do the job:

- The swimming pool industry

  - National Spa and Pool Institute (NSPI)
  - National Swimming Pool Foundation (NSPF)

- Governmental agencies

  - U.S. Consumer Product Safety Commission (CPSC)
  - National Park Service
  - Army Corps of Engineers
  - U.S. Forest Service

- Professional organizations, such as

  - American Red Cross (ARC)
  - National Safety Council (NSC)
  - American Alliance for Health, Physical Education, Recreation, and Dance (AAHPERD) Aquatics Council
  - National Recreation and Park Association (NRPA), Aquatics Section
  - National Water Safety Congress
  - National Aquatic Coalition
  - United States Diving (USD)
  - United States Swimming (USS)
  - YMCA/YWCA

- Media

  - Commercial television production companies
  - Public television producers
  - National media advertisement firms and council

- Educational institutions and organizations

  - Colleges and universities, physical education departments, and continuing education divisions
  - School districts and cooperative service boards

  - Architectural, landscape architectural, and engineering fields
  - Building industry

These videos should illustrate the essential elements for executing safe dives into pools and other aquatic settings, and also the features that constitute unsafe dives with a description of the potential consequences. (See the recommendations for a proposed instructional sign (Table 15.1) later in this chapter.)

"Water Safety Week"

Governments at all levels should proclaim a "water safety week" designed to elevate the general public's level of consciousness relative to the dangers associated with the potential for diving and drowning accidents.

Revision of Educational Curricula

All schools, colleges, agencies, public pools, and other facilities where swimming and diving are taught should revise their curricula to include discussions, demonstrations, and instructions concerning the mechanics of safe diving and the actions that may result in spinal cord injuries. In addition, the teaching of essential safety protective maneuvers to be employed in diving must be emphasized.

Communicating Directly with the Potential Diver

Communicate directly with the person who is contemplating a dive into a pool. This is best accomplished by utilizing the following two approaches:

Verbal messages

First, verbally communicate essential safety instructions to pool users, particularly those meeting the profile, and supervise them to make certain that they follow the instructions and directions. Lifeguards can do this best.

Posted pool rules and warning signs

Second, post clear, concise rules at the entrances that describe the behavior and activities allowed and disallowed in and around the pool. If diving is to be prohibited in certain areas of the pool, adequate warning signs must then be posted at the precise locations of that prohibition. (See Chapter 13 and Appendix A.)

Urgent Need to Inform

Because the risk of spinal cord injury does not appear to be widely understood, an urgency exists to inform patrons of the danger. An adequate warning could reasonably be expected to alter conduct. Absent that preexisting knowledge of the danger, the warning must instruct about the danger as well as warn against it. In either event, and in some other circumstances, unmistakable prohibition should not be the only solution.

The attitude among pool industry people that consistently underestimates the tools of warning as a major accident prevention device must change. Specifically, it is the low level of safety consciousness of individual members of the pool industry that dictates the need to establish standards for pool builders, owners, and operators. (See Appendix A.)

Increasing Responsibility of Pool Builders, Owners, and Operators

The people who design and manufacture swimming pools, both the aboveground and package pools, and those who plan beaches can and must design them so that they are safer. Similarly, those who own pools and beaches, particularly the homeowners and motel/hotel and apartment/condominium owners where approximately 90% of the injuries occur, can and must manage and operate them in a safer manner.

Considerable responsibility falls on the shoulders of homeowners who have little, if any, specialized knowledge concerning diving injuries. They need special guidance targeted at ensuring the safe operation of their own pools and surrounding environment (see Appendix A). To achieve this, these four steps must be taken:

- Support aquatic education and instruction of the public by every means possible.
- Communicate with users of pools and beaches through warning and instructional signs.
- Inspect aquatic areas and facilities on a regular basis.
- Provide an adequate number of qualified lifeguards and supervisors to ensure the safety of patrons.

Regulate Swimming Pools and Beaches

There is the need for better regulation of swimming pools and beaches. There is no question that we have arrived at the time when swimming pools need stronger industry standards and governmental laws and regulations with respect to their design and method of operation. Currently, the pool industry (NSPI) and the American Public Health Association (APHA) are the only two agencies that have provided any guidance for residential pool builders and manufacturers. Both have failed to adequately address the problem of pool safety.

No state at the present time has produced any regulations governing residential pools. States, or at least cities, will have to begin to provide some kind of guidance, if not regulations, for the design and operation of residential pools. Additionally, all 50 states must review their current regulations governing public pools to strengthen these facilities in the area of safety. Some states are improving their safety regulations based on new research. Unfortunately, other states are actually softening their regulations for supervision of semipublic pools in response to pressures from the hotel, motel, and apartment industries. The pressures applied by these industries are misplaced. There are no real economies to be achieved at the expense of safety.

Better state laws and regulations are needed to regulate the design and operation of swimming beaches operated by cities, counties, and commercial enterprises such as resort hotels, motels, and water theme parks, including such examples as:

- Horizontal limits of beaches
- Vertical limits of beaches
- Slope of bottom
- Diving areas
- Nonswimming areas
- Type and location of lifelines
- Erosion prevention
- Water quality
- Signage (beach rules and warning signs)

STANDARDS FOR BOAT DOCKS

Some types of standards, or at least guidelines, need to be developed to regulate the design, installation, and operation of both private and public boat docks, launching ramps, floats, and piers. Such specifications should address the height and width of docks, need for depth markers, and signs prohibiting diving because in most cases the water is not deep enough to safely accommodate diving. These all need to be addressed because it is apparent that many of the injuries occurring each year in the natural environment are the result of people diving from structures extending into lakes, rivers, and oceans.

NEED FOR ADDITIONAL RESEARCH

The need for additional research and, in some instances, continuation of current research, is crucial for increasing the knowledge of how, where, and to whom these diving injuries occur. This should provide the basis for improving the safe design and operation of pools. Additionally, the handling and medical treatment of victims need to be continuously studied. Some of the research needed involves the topics and examples that are listed next.

Human Performance of Divers

The human performance analysis of divers is necessary to determine the following:

- Entry velocity of divers performing from different types of boards
- Entry point of divers
- Distance various types of springboards and jumpboards project divers out from boards of different sizes and heights from the water
- Height divers can achieve from various types of boards
- Trajectory of divers
- Body alignment of divers
- Deceleration rate of divers
- Methods of arresting diver's speed underwater
- Relative position of hands, arms, and head during trajectory
- Head alignment with the body
- Force placed on divers' arms and head at various depths in the pool
- Maximum force divers can arrest by the strength of the arms
- Effect of the slipperiness of the bottom of the pool basin on reducing protection capabilities of arms to absorb the shock of striking the bottom

Warning Signs and Pool Rules

The human factors analysis of warning signs and pool rules (see Chapter 13) is necessary to determine the following:

- Content, size, and location of signs in pools warning against diving
- Content, size, and location of rules governing the use of pools by patrons
- Effectiveness of various types of warning signs and pool rules

Pool and Its Equipment

The pool and its equipment need investigation to determine:

- Methods that may be employed to delineate the contour of the bottom of pools to improve the visibility
- Specifications of the pool diving envelope required to safely accommodate diving from springboards and jumpboards of various sizes
- Performance qualities of the designs of various stands and fulcrums used in conjunction with noncompetitive springboards and jumpboards
- Minimum and desirable levels of in-water and area lighting required for safe swimming and diving at night and indoors
- Safe location of swimming pools with respect to the distance from adjacent structures
- Safe coefficient of friction of vinyl liners used in pools as the water container
- Best color or combination of colors for high visibility of pool basins

Effects of Alcohol and Drugs

It is necessary to determine the effects of alcohol and drugs on diving as well as diving performance. Because 46% of the injuries recorded in this book were alcohol related, a study is needed.

Development of a Data Set and Database System

Database development is necessary to establish a standard system for collecting, recording, analyzing, and reporting data on all spinal cord or head injuries resulting from diving into swimming pools and other water bodies. All these data are essential for facilitating research.

THE DILEMMA

As we begin the new millennium, the swimming pool industry and all those who design, build, sell, own, and operate swimming pools are confronted with the following dilemma—should all diving into water that is 5-ft deep or less be prohibited?

This would apply to not only dives into swimming pools but also those from docks and piers extending into lakes and oceans. As the authors of this book, we feel compelled to take a position on this highly controversial issue and recommend a potentially successful prevention program.

We say absolutely no to those who recommend the prohibition of all diving into water depths of 5 ft or less and to those who even go so far as to say that the safe depth is 9 ft deep. We believe that people should be permitted to dive once they have learned how to do a safe, shallow dive.

People breaking their necks by diving into pools became evident in the 1960s. As a result, those who were injured began to sue the designers, sellers, installers, and owners of pools. Two important facts surfaced through these suits. First, the pool diving envelope designed to provide a safe area for dives off springboards and jumpboards was faulty and dangerous. Second, the supervision of pool patrons by pool owners and operators was practically nonexistent.

The public learned about these diving accidents through newspaper accounts and national TV programs. The first national TV programs that addressed the diving injury problem were on CBS and ABC in 1982. Since then, at least five additional national TV shows on the subject of diving injuries have been televised—"Inside Edition" (three shows), "CBS 60 Minutes," and several local TV presentations. These shows and the many local newspaper accounts of diving accidents elevated the concern of the pool industry, and those who own and operate swimming pools.

Diving, in our opinion, is without question the most exciting and fun activity people can do in a pool; furthermore, they will continue to dive regardless of the signs that say "no diving," because they have been taught how to dive safely in shallow water. At the beginning of the new millennium, the number of diving injuries occurring in pools has been sharply reduced, by as much as 50%. This reduction stems largely from better control of swimmers using pools and lakes, and by the posting of warning signs. However, without doubt, another important factor in this reduction is the intervention of insurance companies that have instructed owners of pools to remove springboards and jumpboards from their pools and to post signs prohibiting diving in the shallow portion.

The signs produced to warn people about diving into the pool have proven to be only partly successful. Consequently, we believe the next step in the process of informing people contemplating a dive is to instruct them how to do so safely in shallow water (3 to 5 ft). This, we believe, can be accomplished by a worded sign that instructs the potential diver what he/she must do to make a safe dive. An example of such a sign is provided in Table 15.1. After the sign we recommend the inclusion of three pictorials (either photos or drawings) that would make it more meaningful by illustrating the following aspects of diving:

- Correct body position for start of dive from the deck of pool or dock
- Proper body alignment of diver above water
- Underwater body position in a shallow dive

This is the dilemma confronting all those who design, own, and operate pools, particularly those who publish standards (NSPI) and produce the laws and regulations governing the design and operation of pools. The reasoning for our decision not to prohibit diving in pools includes:

1. There are now an estimated 250 spinal cord injuries resulting in quadriplegia that occur annually from dives into swimming pools with 20% of them resulting from dives off springboards and jumpboards.
2. Assuming that in the year 2000 there are approximately 6 million active, operating, swimming pools in the United States, and that one dive was made in each pool each day, the total number of dives would be 6 million. If, on the other hand, six dives were made in each pool, the total number for one day would be 36 million. (Some public pools have significantly more dives, while some residential pools may have no dives made at all.) At that rate, there would be an estimated 3 billion, 240 million dives made in pools during, the three summer months. Assuming that there were 180 quadriplegics produced in that period, it would mean approximately 2 a day.

TABLE 15.1
Sample Instructional Sign

You Must Read and Follow These Instructions Before Diving into the Pool

1. You must plan where and how you will dive.
2. Do standing dives only from the deck of the pool (Figure 15.1a). Never run and dive.
3. Pick a spot about 6 ft in front and dive toward it. Enter the water at an angle from 10 to 15 degrees as shown in Figure 15.1b.
4. Immediately on entry into the water raise your head up, arch your back, and push down with your hands (Figure 15c).
5. If you dive incorrectly (too deep) you can break your neck by hitting the bottom.
6. If you have consumed any alcohol or drugs, do not dive.
7. Remember, once you enter the water unless you alter your direction you can strike the bottom in 3 to 4 tenths of a second at a speed that can break your neck.

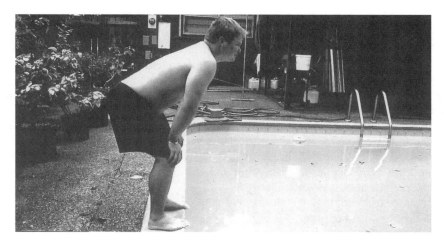

FIGURE 15.1A Correct body position for dive from deck of pool.

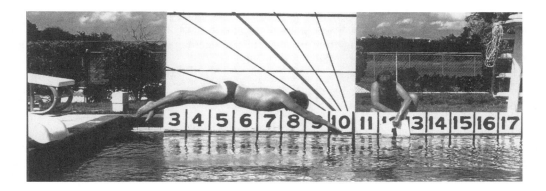

FIGURE 15.1B Correct body alignment above water.

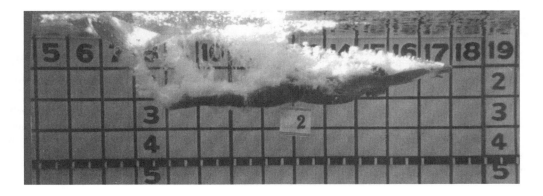

FIGURE 15.1C Correct underwater angle of body in shallow water.

3. The average age of the 440 victims recorded in this book was 23.6 for males and 18.2 for females. There were no children below the age of 12 recorded in the data.

4. Of the 440 accidents, 365(83.0%) happened in these types of pools: residential (228, 51.8%), motel/hotel (72, 16.4%) and apartment/condominium (65, 14.8%). These pools rarely have lifeguards or proper supervision of pool bathers.

5. Of the 440 cases reported in this book, 372(84.5%) occurred in water 5 ft and under with 290(65.9%) in water depths of $3\frac{1}{2}$ ft or less.

6. As the data indicated, males between 18 and 25 were at greatest risk, and children are not at the same level of risk as adults or teenagers.

7. Of the 440 pool-related diving accidents, 179(40.7%) of those injured had consumed some form of alcoholic beverage, mostly beer, and only 7(1.6%) admitted to having taken drugs on the day of the accident.

8. We believe that people will continue to dive into pools regardless of signs being posted saying, "No diving in pool." For pool owners and operators to help eliminate or at least reduce the number of injuries resulting from diving off the decks of pools, we believe that warning signs and other methods of conveying information to potential divers must be improved.

No doubt some pool patrons will read and follow the instructions contained in the proposed sign (see Table 15.1) and others will ignore them. We and all others related to the aquatic industry, however, must continue to try every way possible to eliminate or at least reduce the number of these catastrophic injuries resulting from diving into the shallow end of the pool. This implies better signs and visual instructions on how to dive safely.

CONCLUSIONS

It is the opinion of the authors and the Editorial Board that the low level of public appreciation of the risks associated with diving into shallow water greatly increases the responsibility of every person and enterprise engaged in aquatics to practice and promote accident prevention and safety engineering. Until the public is educated, the awareness of the individual concerning diving will remain at the same level as it now exists. In this context, it is lamentable that the public will unwisely continue to conclude that the injured diver "was fooling around."

Generally, an individual is not able to properly recognize the hazards, evaluate the risks, or appreciate the danger involved in diving. This conclusion should sound an ominous chord to all those within the swimming pool industry, sports and recreation personnel, owners of pools, and regulatory bodies. It is unconscionable for them to have the access and means to know better but to do nothing.

The authors and the Editorial Board believe in the principle that any death or serious injury is unacceptable when reasonable means can be used to either prevent death or minimize injury. The test of reasonableness is merely to ascertain if it is technologically and economically feasible to employ accident prevention techniques. Clearly, warning signs and supervision pass that test.

The authors and members of the Editorial Board associated with this book have used the tools of many professions to examine the data and causes of these paralyzing injuries produced by diving. With a deep sense of purpose we offer this book with the hope it may have an impact on those in positions of responsibility so that the number of these catastrophic injuries may be significantly reduced.

Appendix A

This appendix contains documents applicable to the safe operation and management of swimming pools. It also includes the profiles of the accident victims and of the accident pools in the 440 diving injuries. The contents are as follows:

1. Safety checklist for owners, managers, and operators of swimming pools
2. Profile of the diving accident victim
3. Profile of the diving accident pool
4. Suggested rules for use of aboveground pools
5. Activities that should be prohibited in aboveground pools
6. What every operator of public and semipublic pools should do to ensure the safety of patrons
7. Instructions for the use of the pool to be given to tenants and guests of apartments/condominiums
9. What every motel/hotel owner/operator should do to maximize the safety of their pool guests
10. What every apartment/condominium owner/operator should do to maximize the safety of pool users

SAFETY CHECKLIST FOR OWNERS, MANAGERS, AND OPERATORS OF SWIMMING POOLS

This checklist is for use by anyone who has any connection with the management and operation of swimming pools. The safe operation of a pool is complex and requires constant attention. Although this checklist is primarily directed at public and semipublic pools, many of the items apply to owners of residential pools as well.

Yes	No		
		1.	Are you familiar with your state regulations governing public and semipublic pools?
		2.	Are you familiar with local regulations and building codes applicable to your pool?
		3.	Are you familiar with the National Spa and Pool Institute (NSPI) and the U.S. Consumer Product Safety Commission (CPCS) that have safety materials available on the operation of pools?
		4.	Have you achieved a personal level of knowledge of the procedures essential to the safe operation of your pool?
		5.	Have you established, in writing, the safety policies and procedures governing the operation of your pool?
		6.	Does your policy establish who else within your staff must be qualified in CPR and first aid procedures other than your lifeguards?
		7.	Do you have qualified lifeguards assigned to your pool to provide for the supervision of patrons or guests?
		8.	Have you, as owner or manager of a pool, ensured that instructions for the use of the pool are given to your guests?
		9.	Do you have "Rules for Pool Use" posted at each pool entrance?
		10.	Do you have warnings on the deck at the edge of the pool prohibiting diving in areas where the water is less than 5' deep?
		11.	Have you made provisions for accommodating disabled people (i.e. those in wheelchairs) who wish to use your pool?
		12.	Do you have a qualified pool operator to inspect the pool and equipment every day to ensure that they are in good operating condition?
		13.	Is your pool presently equipped with the essential first aid, life support, and lifeguard equipment, including a spineboard?
		14.	Does your pool have the legally required and necessary lifesaving equipment mounted on appropriate stands in the immediate area of the pool?
		15.	Do you have a telephone located within the pool area with the emergency telephone numbers listed?
		16.	Have you established a plan to handle common emergencies and accidents that may occur in your pool?
		17.	Have you established a system for recording and reporting accidents that happen in the pool?
		18.	Does your pool have a proper barrier around it, with a self-closing, self-latching gate or door, which will prevent access to the pool when it is officially closed?
		19.	Have you established on-site security personnel or a means of surveillance of the pool via TV monitors and/or pool alarms when the pool is closed?

		20.	If you have a springboard installed, does your pool have a safe diving envelope, with sufficientb depth of water in the diving well to safely accommodate its size and height?
		21.	If your pool has a water slide, does it meet the suggested standards of the U.S. CPCS?
		22.	If your pool has a spa or hot tub, do you have a cover for it that will prevent access to it when it is closed?
		23.	Have you established a safety checklist for assessing the need for the annual repair or replacement of equipment, especially at the end of the pool season?
		24.	Do you budget for equipment replacements as needed and for periodic repair and repainting of the pool?
		25.	Are you aware of the high risk of aquatic activities that your patrons or guests may participate in?
		26.	Have you ever had a risk management assessment of your pool performed by a professional safety expert?
		27.	Do you carry adequate accident and liability insurance to cover any injury occurring in your pool?
		28.	As owner of a residential pool, do you assign an adult (or employ a lifeguard) to supervise your guests when you have a pool party where ten or more people are in attendance?
		29.	Do you know about the dangers confronting people who are intoxicated, and the appropriateness of prohibiting them from using the pool?
		30.	Do you have written pool closing procedures, used on a daily basis, to ensure that the pool was closed and witnessed by a staff member, without leaving someone behind?

PROFILE OF THE DIVING ACCIDENT VICTIM

This profile is compiled from the study of 440 pool diving accidents.

- The victim was a male of an average age of 24. (Females were 18.1.)
- He was close to 6 ft in height and weighed over 175 lb.
  (Females were 5 ft 6 in. in height and weighed 124 lb.)
- He taught himself to dive, with no formal diving instruction.
- He was not aware that he could break his neck making a dive where he did.
- He was visiting the pool for the first time as a guest, and the dive he made when injured was the first one made in that pool.
- He was performing a shallow dive with his hands in front when entering the water.
- He had witnessed other people diving into the pool before making the catastrophic dive.
- He was not warned—either by verbal instructions or by signs—to refrain from diving at the place of his accident or into shallow water less than 5 ft in depth.
- He struck the bottom of the pool as opposed to the pool sidewall.
- He did not lose consciousness after striking the bottom and only sustained a slight abrasion and/or laceration to the apex of the head.
- He was removed from the pool by friends who were not aware that he had fractured his neck. No spineboard was used.
- He was not intoxicated, according to witnesses.
- He had not used drugs the preceding 24 h.
- His injury was a compression fracture of the cervical spine at the level of C-5 or C-5, 6.
- He was diagnosed by doctors as a quadriplegic and paralyzed for life.

PROFILE OF THE DIVING ACCIDENT POOL

This profile was taken from the study of 440 pool diving accidents.

- The pool was typically owned and operated by a homeowner, motel/hotel, or apartment/condominium.
- The operator of the pool was not aware of the dangers related to diving into a swimming pool.
- No lifeguard was on duty at the pool at the time of the accident.
- When dives were made from the pool deck, the water depth where the victim struck the bottom was less than 4 ft.
- When the victim made a dive from a springboard or jumpboard, the victim impacted the bottom at the transition between the deep and shallow portion of the pool (upslope) where the depth of water was less than 6 ft.
- The water was turbid (cloudy) or semiturbid in 60% of the pools, making it difficult to clearly discern the bottom.
- The lighting, both in the pool and in the pool surroundings, was below acceptable standards in the accidents that occurred at night.
- There were no warning signs prohibiting diving.
- There were no bottom or depth markings in the pool.
- There was an absence of lifesaving and emergency equipment and procedures.
- The general environment of the pool created an illusion of safety.

SUGGESTED RULES FOR USE OF ABOVEGROUND POOLS

Rules for use of this pool follow—(for your safety please obey them):

- Do not dive. This is a shallow, constant depth swimming pool with an overall depth of $3\frac{1}{2}$ ft.
- It is dangerous to dive in this pool.
- If you choose to dive, you can suffer a serious or fatal injury.
- Enter and leave the pool only by means of the ladder.
- Horseplay of any kind is not permitted—pushing or throwing people into the pool is prohibited.
- If you have consumed any alcohol, do not use the pool.
- Swimming alone is dangerous and, therefore, prohibited.
- Children must never be left alone in or around the pool, not even for seconds.
- Do not use the pool if an electrical storm is approaching.
- Do not swim at night unless underwater and overhead pool lights are in use.
- Do not use glassware in or around the pool.

ACTIVITIES THAT SHOULD BE PROHIBITED IN ABOVEGROUND POOLS

PROHIBIT DIVES FROM THE DECK

- Any dive from the deck, ladder, or pool seat (rim)
- Running dives from the deck
- Back dives from the deck or rim of the pool
- Diving through inner tubes or hula hoops
- Diving from a jumpboard or trampoline placed on the deck
- Diving through the legs of people standing in the pool

PROHIBIT DIVES ORIGINATING FROM OUTSIDE THE POOL

- Running in the yard and diving over the rim into the pool
- Diving from adjacent structures (porch, garage, etc.)
- Diving from a trampoline on the ground outside of the pool
- Diving from a slide into the pool

PROHIBIT THESE OTHER ACTIVITIES

- Somersaulting into the pool
- Going down a slide outside of the pool with an exit into the pool
- Going down a slide placed on the deck
- Handspring from a run in the yard, placing hands on the rim
- Games such as "Marco Polo" or "follow the leader" that might involve diving
- Pushing people into the pool from the deck
- Throwing people into the pool from the deck or from outside the pool
- Swinging into the pool from a rope attached to a tree
- Jumping or diving from a trampoline

REMEMBER, SAFETY IS NO ACCIDENT

WHAT EVERY OPERATOR OF PUBLIC AND SEMIPUBLIC POOLS SHOULD DO TO ENSURE THE SAFETY OF PATRONS

- Provide a certified lifeguard on duty at all times when the pool is open for use.
- Install a 6-ft-high fence with self-closing, self-latching gates capable of being locked.
- Post signs at every entrance stating the rules for the use of the pool.
- Post signs prohibiting diving in areas of the pool where the water is less than 5 ft deep, and in other areas where diving is dangerous.
- Provide accurate depth markers both on the interior wall above the water line and on the coping or edge of the pool.
- Mark the bottom of the pool to enable a person contemplating a dive to visualize the pool bottom.
- Adequate lighting conforming to (IES), American Public Health Association (APHA), or state standards both in the interior and the surrounding area if the pool is to be used at night.
- Where springboards are provided for competitive diving, the water depth and bottom configuration must conform to the design specifications promulgated by the ruling bodies (United States Diving [USD], National Collegiate Athletic Association [NCAA], and National Federation of State High School, Athletic Associations, [NFSHSAA]).
- Pools with diving equipment not used for competition should be limited to boards no longer than 10 ft, with a depth of water at the plummet of 10 ft, and extending forward for 16 ft before the start of the upslope (see Figure 12.2.)

INSTRUCTIONS FOR THE USE OF THE POOL TO BE GIVEN
TO TENANTS AND GUESTS OF APARTMENTS/CONDOMINIUMS

- The swimming pool has been provided for your enjoyment as well as your family and guests.
- Please read and obey the following rules that apply to the use of the pool.

GENERAL INFORMATION

- There is no lifeguard on duty.
- Do not use the pool alone.
- Positively no swimming is allowed when the pool is closed.
- When entering the pool for the first time, walk around, read all signs, and identify the depth of the pool by observing depth markers, as well as the location of emergency equipment including the telephone.
- Enter the pool the first time by going down the steps or ladder in the shallow end of the pool and walk around to familiarize yourself with the depth, slope of the bottom, etc.
- Do not bring breakable objects (i.e., glassware) to the pool.
- Do not use the pool if you have been drinking alcoholic beverages.
- People with skin, ear, or other infections should not use the pool.
- No dogs or cats are allowed in the pool area.
- Get out of the pool if lightning is in the area.
- No horseplay, running on the deck, pushing, or throwing people in the pool are permitted.
- No walking or playing is allowed on the wall separating the children's pool from the main pool.

DIVING

- Diving into pool is only permitted in the deep end of the pool (depth more than 5 ft).
- If you, or your children, dive into the shallow portion of the pool (under 5 ft), serious or fatal injury may result.
- The use of scuba equipment is prohibited.
- Never dive through inner tubes or hula hoops.

USE BY CHILDREN

- There is no lifeguard on duty. Therefore, you must supervise your children at all times they use the pool. Watching your children by looking out the window of your room is unacceptable.
- If you have to leave the pool for any reason, have your children leave the pool and sit down until you return.
- Do not rely on other adults around the pool to supervise your children.
- Children who are nonswimmers must stay in the wading pool.
- The use of flotation devices, such as rubber rafts and inner tubes, must be carefully supervised.
- For children who need to be helped, throw them the life ring, be sure to hold on to the line, or use the shepherd's crook.

IN AN EMERGENCY

If you see anyone in trouble, sound the alarm that is the red button located by the phone; then dial 911 or the local rescue squad from the from the list of emergency phone numbers.

WHAT EVERY MOTEL/HOTEL OWNER/OPERATOR SHOULD DO TO MAXIMIZE THE SAFETY OF THEIR POOL GUESTS

SUPERVISION

- Provide certified lifeguards at all times the pool is officially open.
- Never place full responsibility on parents to watch their children.

COMMUNICATION

- Communicate with the guests and owners concerning instructions for the safe use of the pool.
- Post pool rules at every entrance to the facility with an emphasis on **no diving** when the pool is not safe for diving.

MARKERS AND SIGNS

- Stencil signs on all sides of the pool indicating the prohibition against diving where the depth of water is less than 5 ft.
- Place depth markers (at least 4 in. high, 6 in. preferred) at the edge of the pool and on the internal wall above the water line in accordance with state regulations.
- Mark all internal steps with a 2-in.-wide stripe on the vertical and horizontal ledges and place a black line 6 in. wide down the center of the longitudinal axis of the pool.

SECURITY

- Make certain the pool can be secured when it is officially closed. This means having a satisfactory barrier around all four sides of the pool with self-closing, self-latching gates capable of being locked. A pool cover can be used for small pools.

POOL DESIGN

- If planning a new pool, be sure the profile of the bottom in the diving portion conforms to the specifications set forth in Figure 12.2.
- Remove the springboard if water depth does not conform to the bottom profile shown in Figure 12.2.
- When planning a pool, make certain it is located at least 20 ft from any structure from which someone might dive, as well as from the children's wading pool, and from the spa or hot tub.
- Never place a 3-m springboard in your pool unless the depth conforms to regulations for competitive diving by NCAA or USD, which is a minimum of 13 ft.

WHAT EVERY APARTMENT/CONDOMINIUM OWNER/ OPERATOR SHOULD DO TO MAXIMIZE THE SAFETY OF POOL USERS

SUPERVISION

* Have qualified, certified lifeguards on duty at all times the pool is officially open.

COMMUNICATION

* Communicate with the tenants and owners concerning instruction for the safe use of the pool as shown in this appendix.
* Post rules at every entrance to the pool with an emphasis on **no diving** when the pool is not safe for diving.

MARKERS AND SIGNS

* Stencil deck markings or signs on all sides of the pool indicating the prohibition of diving where the depth of water is less than 5 ft.
* Place depth markers (at least 4 in. high, 6 in. preferred) at the edge of the pool and on the internal wall above the water line in accordance with state regulations.
* Outline all internal steps with a 2-in.-wide strip on the vertical and horizontal ledges and place a black line 6 in. wide down the center of the longitudinal axis of the pool.

SECURITY

* Make certain the pool can be secured when it is officially closed. This means having a satisfactory barrier around the pool and locks for each gate.
* Install night-lights that activate at twilight if the pool is used for night swimming.
* Utilize a video surveillance camera during normal hours of operation capable of being monitored from the manager's office.

POOL DESIGN

* If planning a new pool, be sure the profile of the bottom in the diving portion conforms to the specification.
* Remove the springboard if water depth does not conform to state regulations.
* When planning a pool, make certain it is located a safe distance from any structure, as well as from the children's wading pool and from the spa or hot tub.

Appendix B*

Photographs contained in this appendix (Figures B.1 through B.16) illustrate divers performing off springboards/jumpboards and slides, and from the deck of the pool located on the campus of Nova Southeastern University, Fort Lauderdale, Florida. The dive/slide research pool was constructed in 1972 for the purpose of conducting research on diving and sliding. The specifications of the pool are 30 × 36 ft in size, 12 ft deep overall, with an underwater room having a window to permit photographs of divers underwater. The above water and underwater grids consist of lines 12 in. in size. The video and still cameras are 24 ft from the subjects performing the dives. Figures B.3 through B.16 show divers both above and below the surface of the water doing different types of dives. Above water and in-water speeds were calculated and are covered in Chapter 10. The photographs depicted here are

- Figures B.1 and B.2: Photos of the Dive/Slide Research Center showing the above water and underwater grids
- Figures B.3 and B.4: Photos showing the diver's entry point into the pool, from dives off recreational-type boards
- Figures B.5 and B.6: Photos showing the diver underwater with the head about to intersect with the simulated bottom profile of a pool at a water depth of 4 to 5 ft and a distance of 15 and 18 ft from the end of the springboard
- Figures B.7 and B.8: Showing recreational divers actually overshooting the pool diving envelope as indicated by the dotted line
- Figures B.9 and B.10: In bottom photo showing diver steering up; and in top photo the diver about to interact with the bottom (dotted line) 18 ft from the end of the board
- Figures B.11 and B.12: Depicting shallow dives from the deck
- Figures B.13 and B.14: Depicting underwater shots of shallow-water dives
- Figures B.15 and B.16: Showing competitive divers performing off 3-m-high springboard at the International Swimming Hall of Fame diving pool

---

* Photos taken at Dive/Slide Research Facility at Nova Southeastern University, Ft. Lauderdale, Florida.

Photos that follow depict the Dive/Slide Research Facility at Nova Southeastern University in Fort Lauderdale, Florida.

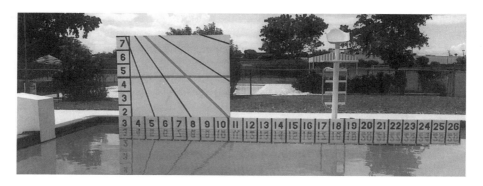

FIGURE B.1   The above water grid.

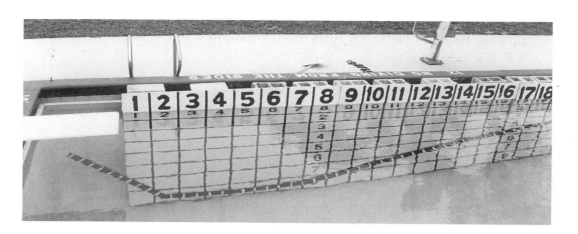

FIGURE B.2   The underwater grid.